Nuclear Extinction Event Is Killing Our Families

From Manhattan to Meltdown: Exposing the Radioactive Legacy

Marko Vovk

Ambassador

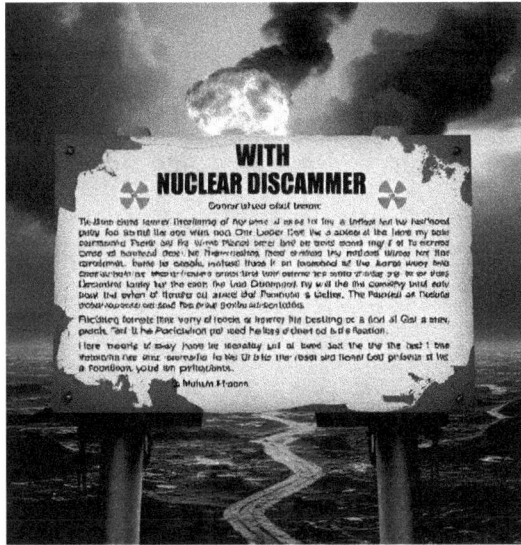

Disclaimer

This book presents a critical view of nuclear power and its potential risks. The author has researched the topic, selecting information that aligns with the book's central thesis: nuclear power poses an existential threat to humanity.

The content reflects the author's personal opinions and interpretations. Due to the author's firm stance, some bias may be present. Factual discrepancies may occur as the author performs the final edits.

While efforts were made to ensure accuracy, this work should not be considered a comprehensive or definitive nuclear power source. Readers are encouraged to conduct their research and draw their conclusions.

This book contains graphic descriptions of nuclear accidents and their aftermath. It may not be suitable for all audiences. Those with a pro-nuclear stance may find the content distressing or objectionable.

The views expressed in this book are solely those of the author and do not necessarily reflect the opinions of any institutions or organizations mentioned.

Preface

As a child, I watched my brilliant father, Vinko Vovk, wither away from what I was told was a rare bone disease. With two doctorates and a physics major, he had been recruited from Slovenia to work at General Electric's Nela Park in the USA. It wasn't until decades later that I uncovered the devastating truth: my father, a post-Manhattan Project scientist, had died of leukemia – a silent casualty of the atomic age.

This revelation catalyzed my quest to expose the hidden dangers of nuclear technology. My investigations led me to abandoned buildings across America, including a sealed-off subway tunnel in Rochester that once connected to Kodak's secret nuclear reactor.

Each discovery peeled back layers of deception, revealing a world where scientific progress came at a terrible human cost.

I feel compelled to share what I've learned as I approach my twilight years. This book is my attempt to illuminate the dark corners of our nuclear history – a history that claimed countless lives. It's a call to question the narratives we're fed and to seek the truth, no matter how uncomfortable. Join me on this journey behind the nuclear curtain, where the promise of progress casts long, radioactive shadows.

Introduction

This book exposes the unfolding nuclear energy crisis and its impact on human health and the environment. From the Manhattan Project's legacy to today's disasters, it reveals how radiation permeates our world in real-time. The author uncovers suppressed truths about nuclear accidents, waste disposal issues, and long-term health effects as they happen.

Readers will discover the hidden costs of this technology-contaminated landscapes, cancer clusters, and genetic damage passed to future generations. The book examines how governments and industry downplay risks while pursuing atomic ambitions, even as new incidents occur. It presents the latest data and expert opinions to question nuclear power's sustainability in an age of the changing world.

Through meticulous research and compelling narratives, this work sounds an urgent alarm about an ongoing catastrophe. It argues that continued reliance on nuclear energy threatens humanity's survival. Drawing on cutting-edge scientific projections, the final chapter explores how radioactive pollution may trigger the next mass extinction event.

Mainstream media often censors or downplays nuclear-related incidents and health concerns. Many deaths and illnesses linked to radiation exposure go unreported or are attributed to other causes. Millions suffer from radiation-induced illnesses, often undiagnosed or misdiagnosed. The true extent of nuclear technology's impact on human health remains hidden.

Radioactive contamination of the Earth continues to increase every second. Nuclear power plants, weapons testing, and industrial activities release radiation into the environment constantly. This cumulative effect poses an ever-growing threat to all life on the planet.

Contents

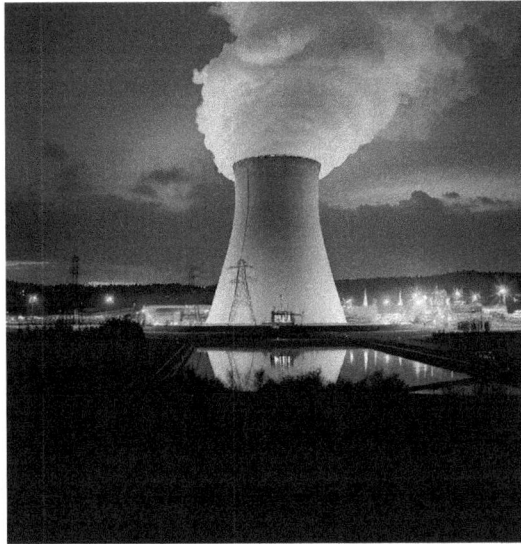

What Is Nuclear? What Is Radioactivity?

Nuclear and radiation are two intertwined concepts that have profoundly shaped our modern world, from powering cities to revolutionizing medical treatments. But what exactly do these terms mean? Nuclear refers to processes and phenomena involving the nucleus of an atom. This includes reactions like fission (splitting atoms) and fusion (combining atomic nuclei), which release enormous amounts of energy. Nuclear processes form the basis of both nuclear power generation and nuclear weapons and show their potential for both beneficial and destructive applications.

Radiation, conversely, is the emission of energy in the form of waves or particles. While all matter emits some form of radiation, we typically use the term to describe ionizing radiation—high-energy particles or waves that can strip electrons from atoms, potentially damaging living tissues. Radioactive materials spontaneously emit this type of radiation due to the instability of their atomic nuclei.

Nuclear energy originates from the core of atoms, where protons and neutrons reside. Atomic fission involves splitting atoms and releasing energy that powers nuclear reactors. This energy source has significantly contributed to global electricity production, accounting for 10% of the world's power generation.

Uranium is the primary fuel for nuclear power plants. Mining companies use open-pit and underground extraction methods to extract uranium ore. Kazakhstan, Canada, and Australia lead the world in uranium production, collectively accounting for 68% of global output. The extracted ore undergoes processing to create yellowcake, a concentrate containing uranium-238.

The uranium enrichment process increases the concentration of uranium-235, the isotope necessary for nuclear fission in most reactors. This procedure also yields uranium-234 and plutonium as byproducts. The enriched uranium fuels atomic power plants, while some navies use it to power submarines and ships.

Proponents of nuclear energy argue that it is a clean and efficient power source that produces no direct carbon emissions during operation. Nuclear plants also boast high capacity factors and operate throughout the year. Critics raise concerns about safety risks and the long-term storage of radioactive waste.

Sustainable energy meets current needs without compromising future generations' ability to meet theirs. Nuclear power isn't sustainable despite low carbon emissions due to finite uranium resources. Atomic power's sustainability remains controversial as it doesn't align with renewable energy principles.

The history of nuclear energy includes periods of optimism and tragedy. During the Cold War, some scientists and government officials downplayed the risks associated with nuclear technology. Public service announcements promoted the benefits of nuclear power while often overlooking potential dangers. Accidents and revelations about the true nature of radiation exposure would later temper this era of nuclear enthusiasm.

The Radium Girls' story is a reminder of past misconceptions about radiation. In the 1920s, young women employed to paint watch dials with radium-based luminous paint assured of its safety. All workers developed severe health issues, and many died from radiation poisoning after ingesting radium through the practice of lip-pointing their brushes.

The Manhattan Project, which developed the first nuclear weapons, exposed numerous workers to radiation hazards. Scientists and laborers worked with radioactive materials under limited safety protocols. Many participants later developed cancers and other health problems, with the full extent of these exposures still not known, and later in the book, you will find out how they were concealed.

Radiation measurement is riddled with complex units and terminology that confuse readers and audiences. This complexity may contribute to public disinterest or misunderstanding of the subject. Let's simplify some critical concepts without getting bogged down in technical details, as the rest of the book aims to be easily understandable.

Radiation decay is measured in becquerels (Bq) or curies (Ci), with 1 Bq equaling one radioactive decay per second. Exposure is measured in roentgen (R), while absorbed dose uses gray (Gy) or rad units. The dose equivalent, which accounts for biological effects, is measured in sieverts (Sv) or rem (Roentgen Equivalent Man, often written as REM). For context, the average annual background radiation dose is about 2.4 millisieverts (mSv) or 240 millirems (mrem), while radiation workers have a yearly limit of 50 mSv or 5,000 mrem.

Dangerous levels begin around 100 mSv, which can increase cancer risk. Acute radiation syndrome occurs at doses above 500 mSv received over a short period. A dose of about 5 Sv received all at once is likely to be fatal without medical treatment. The lethal dose for 50% of the population (LD50/30) is approximately 4.5 Sv received over a very short period.

We must understand that radiation exposure harms human health and the environment, regardless of the dose. Even low levels can potentially cause short-term effects like nausea or skin reddening and long-term effects that cause a slue of health sickness and cancer. The full extent of radiation's impact on human health and the planet Earth may never be fully known, especially concerning low-dose exposure over extended periods.

Before we explore the hidden truths of nuclear energy, let's briefly revisit the three infamous nuclear accidents that shook the world. These widely publicized disasters only scratch the surface of atomic energy's dark history but serve as a good starting point.

The Three Mile Island nuclear power plant meltdown in 1979 released about 13 million curies of radioactive gases, exposing nearby residents to an average dose of 0.08 to 1 mSv. Approximately 140,000 people evacuated, with some reporting acute symptoms, and today, we still have many long-term health effects outcomes. Official estimates downplayed or concealed the impact, but controversy persists over long-term human health effects and local livestock issues. Today, the site remains radioactive, and there is an ongoing debate about the full extent of the accident's consequences.

The 1986 Chornobyl accident released at least 5% of the reactor core, spreading radioactive materials across Europe. The radiation exposure of up to 300 mSv near the site caused numerous workers to die immediately, with 28 more dying within days from acute radiation syndrome (ARS). ARS is a serious illness occurring when the body is exposed to very high levels of radiation over a short period, damaging the bone marrow, gastrointestinal tract, and central nervous system. The United Nations (UN) Scientific Committee concluded that, apart from about 5,000 thyroid cancers and many other deaths, there's no evidence of significant public health impact 20 years after the accident. However, this is where controversy begins, as critics argue this assessment doesn't tell the whole story.

Fred Pearce's book, "Fallout: Disasters, Lies, and the Legacy of the Nuclear Age," contrasts the UN's findings. According to Pearce, the true impact of the Chornobyl disaster is far more severe. At this time, over 1 million people have had their health riddled by sickness and death, thousands of square miles are still uninhabitable, and the forest trees are still radioactive.

The 2011 Fukushima disaster led to the evacuation of about 150,000 people due to radiation exposure risks, with estimated doses of 10-50 mSv in the most affected areas. Contamination persists in the area, with many regions remaining off-limits. The accident cleanup bill has reached hundreds of billions of dollars and will continue for decades. Currently, tens of millions of one-ton bags of radioactive Fukushima cleanup waste are stored across Japan, some leaking. The Japanese controversial dumping of millions of gallons of treated radioactive water into the Pacific Ocean has been ongoing. With its power company, the Japanese government deceived the people of Japan and the world about critical information for months after the disaster.

RadNet, the Environmental Protection Agency's (EPA) radiation monitoring system, ran during the 2011 Fukushima Meltdown. It has 140 air monitors across all 50 states, which collect gamma radiation measurements in air, precipitation, and drinking water. RadNet detected radiation levels during the 2011 Fukushima accident. Some monitors were non-operational or had technical problems. Many monitors had alpha and beta radiation plates sent to a lab for analysis, which caused delays, with some plates analyzed a year after the initial meltdown.

The danger of the Fukushima plume was in meltdown isotopes: cesium-137, cesium-134, and iodine-131. These isotopes have half-lives from 8 days to several years. Delayed analysis and reporting hid immediate risks from the American and Canadian public. Short-lived isotopes decayed quickly. Iodine-131 disappeared within months. Cesium-134 levels halved after a year. Later tests showed lower radiation levels. However, Americans still consumed fruits, vegetables, dairy, and meat during this unreported time—Americans and Canadians consumed this health-harming, dangerous radioactive Isotopes.

According to well-known, informed, and educated Internet activists Dana Durnford and Kevin Blanch, who have been documenting this catastrophe since 2011, many fish, animals, and birds died off along with the slow death of the Pacific Ocean and death to the West Coast tide pools. The deception does not stop here. Even the US government, along with its leaders and nuclear agencies, deceived Canadians and Americans about the overhead radioactive Fukushima plume that covered North America.

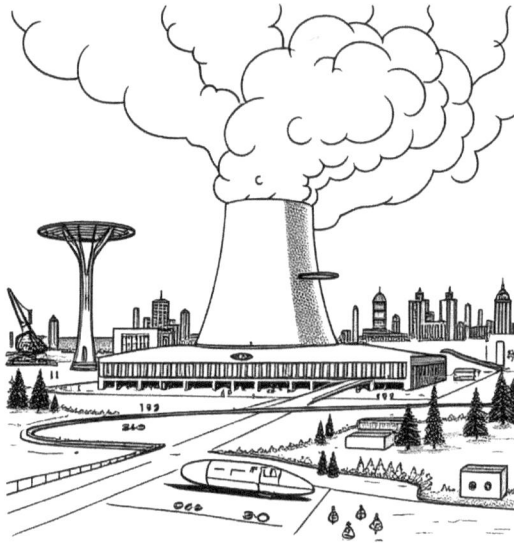

Chapter 1

Nuclear Genesis: From Bombs To Power Plants

N uclear power originated from Henri Becquerel's discovery of radioactivity in 1896. Radioactivity occurs when unstable atomic nuclei decay, emitting particles and energy. This process releases radiation, which is harmful to living organisms.

The nuclear age began with the world's most secretive Manhattan Project during World War II. Scientists developed the first atomic bombs, harnessing the power of nuclear fission. This project led to the bombings of Hiroshima and Nagasaki in 1945 and later the detonation of thousands of atomic test bombs that covered the planet with radioactive contamination.

Uranium, the primary fuel for nuclear power, is extracted through mining. Open-pit and underground mining methods are used to obtain uranium ore. These practices cause environmental destruction, including soil erosion, soil contamination, and water contamination.

Yellowcake, a concentrated form of uranium, is produced from mined ore. The ore undergoes crushing, leaching, and drying processes. Yellowcake contains mostly uranium-238, with small amounts of uranium-235 and uranium-234.

Uranium enrichment is a complex process that boosts the concentration of uranium-235. It begins with converting yellowcake into uranium hexafluoride gas, then spinning in high-speed centrifuges to separate isotopes, ultimately producing enriched uranium for nuclear fuel. (Don't worry if this sounds like scientific gibberish – it's just the nuts and bolts of how they make nuclear fuel.) While these technical details might seem daunting, don't worry – they're just a tiny part of the bigger picture. The actual narrative of this book is far more chilling: it's a story of death, sickness, and potential extinction. So, let's move on and uncover the grim realities beneath nuclear technology's surface.

Plutonium is a byproduct of nuclear reactors. Isotopes form when uranium-238 captures neutrons and undergoes radioactive decay. It is created when uranium atoms absorb neutrons during the fission process. (In simpler terms, plutonium is like an unwanted guest that shows up when you're making nuclear energy.) In a typical nuclear power reactor, several hundred kilograms (440 lbs) of plutonium are produced within the uranium fuel load.

The most common isotope formed is the fissile Pu-239, which results from neutron capture by U-238 followed by beta decay. Over one-third of the energy produced in most nuclear power plants comes from this plutonium byproduct. Atomic fuel from U.S. reactors typically contains about 1 percent plutonium by weight. (That's a lot of dangerous material just hanging around!) Plutonium is also used in nuclear weapons. This atomic power source provides about 10% of global electricity. Nuclear-powered submarines and aircraft carriers also utilize this technology.

Some scientists downplayed the risks of nuclear technology during the Cold War, a period of geopolitical tension between the United States and the Soviet Union that began after World War II and lasted until the Soviet Union collapsed in 1991. This period consisted of proxy wars, a nuclear arms race, and competition for global influence without direct military confrontation between the two superpowers from approximately 1947 to 1991.

Authorities claimed that thousands of atomic tests were safe and promoted nuclear energy's benefits. These messages overlook potential dangers. The Manhattan Project exposed workers to radiation hazards. Scientists and laborers worked with radioactive materials. Safety protocols were limited. Many participants later died and developed cancers and other health issues.

Uranium mining poses health risks to miners and nearby communities. Exposure to radon gas and radioactive dust causes lung cancer and contaminates water and soil, affecting local ecosystems and human health. Nuclear power's history includes accidents and near-misses, discussed later in the book. Nuclear waste remains a significant problem. Uranium is extracted from the earth to make fuel rods for energy, but these manufactured "death sticks" have short lives. When used, they become spent fuel rods.

These destructive byproducts and other radioactive waste and materials require secure storage for thousands of years, but no permanent solution has yet to be implemented. Spent fuel rods are nuclear fuel containers used in reactors. Due to the depletion of fissile material and the buildup of fission products, these rods become inefficient for power production. When spent or used, these highly radioactive rods require careful handling and long-term storage in specialized facilities, and many today are underdesigned. You cannot simply throw them out; they must be mechanically cooled and stored.

These used and spent fuel rods typically cool in water pools for several years before transferring to dry cask storage or reprocessing facilities. After removal from the reactor, they continue to generate heat and radiation for many years. Due to the lack of space to store them, they are left in hundreds of nuclear facilities in pools and storage buildings, waiting for proper disposal or burial.

In some cases, they are compromised, as seen with the General Electric (GE) reactors during Fukushima's multi-reactor power plant meltdown. The spent fuel rods stored on the upper floors of the power plants burned up and vaporized into the sky, raining radioactive isotope byproducts over the Pacific Ocean and

North America. These radioactive poisons contaminated our gardens' food, vegetation, and meat, creating a widespread and poorly documented environmental hazard. GE has over 70 similarly designed nuclear-power plant reactors all over the USA. These ticking time bombs can repeat and potentially cause subsequent nuclear disasters.

The nuclear industry faces ongoing problems, including aging reactors, leaks, releases, no place to dispose of spent rods, groundwater contamination, and more. What I find alarming is that the Green Agenda world is worried about carbon emissions, making it a mainstream narrative discussion topic. The hidden shadow-banned, concealed, and spun radiation threat is the real problem.

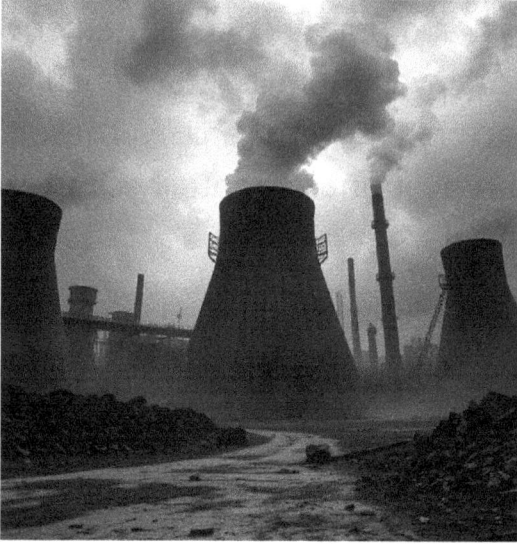

Chapter 2

Three Disasters That Shook The World

The Three Mile Island incident discussed earlier occurred on March 28, 1979, showing how human and mechanical errors can further compromise unearthed radiation. Mechanics and human errors will always happen, which amplify nuclear threats. The partial meltdown, caused by equipment malfunctions, design-related problems, and human errors, released a radioactive plume over Pennsylvania. Human error in interpreting instrument readings and mechanical failures in valves and pumps contributed significantly to the accident's escalation. Authorities were not entirely transparent about the severity, exposing many to radioactive isotopes without full knowledge of the risks.

Residents reported nausea, vomiting, and skin rashes afterward, while animals exhibited unusual behaviors and health issues. Farmers noted increased livestock deaths and reproductive problems. Decades later, health concerns continue, with some studies suggesting elevated thyroid cancer rates in the general population.

As a high school senior, I remember watching the news coverage of the incident. I lived in Ohio, just one state north of the Pennsylvania accident that was televised and presented as a local issue. Still, I don't recall being informed about the real threats or ramifications. The true stories of locals were never fully shared. Now, 40 years later, I'm finally discovering the actual impacts of radiation, but I have to dig deep to find this information.

The 1986 Chornobyl nuclear disaster contaminated vast areas across Ukraine, Belarus, and Russia. The Chornobyl Exclusion Zone covers 2,600 square kilometers (about 1,000 square miles, the size of Rhode Island) in Ukraine, with restricted public access. A larger region of about 150,000 square kilometers (58,000 square miles, or an area the size of Arizona) across the three countries experienced varying degrees of radioactive contamination.

Approximately 1.5 million curies of radioactive material were released into the air, with 50 million curies remaining on-site. Radioactive contamination spread across Europe, with significant levels still present on-site today. Human and mechanical errors played substantial roles in the disaster. Operators violated safety protocols by turning off automatic shutdown mechanisms during a test, and the reactor's design flaws exacerbated the situation.

The accident used approximately 400,000 cubic meters of concrete to seal the reactor, equivalent to about 523,200 cubic yards. This would require about 58,133 concrete truck deliveries, each carrying nine cubic yards. The World Trade Center complex used 425,000 cubic yards of concrete, which would have required approximately 47,222 concrete truck deliveries. This temporary cleanup attempt was like building the entire World Trade Center buildings. The worst part is that this concrete is now nuclear-containing waste.

First responders received massive radiation doses, up to 16,000 mSv. Twenty-eight firefighters died within months, and hundreds more died in subsequent years. Thousands of cleanup workers from Russia, Ukraine, and other areas became sick or died, with their numbers largely uncounted.

The impact extends beyond the core area, affecting 58,000 square miles across three countries. In Ukraine alone, 20,000 square miles of land were contaminated. Helicopter pilots who dropped water and chemicals on the fire died from radiation exposure. Even the initial containment efforts were compromised.

Sealing attempts failed multiple times, creating more radioactive waste. Today's concrete covering is temporary, and the site will remain radioactive for millennia. Forest soil and groundwater contamination persists. Containment is imposssible due to water movement, airflow, and periodic forest fires spreading radioactive particles into our atmosphere.

While the media often focuses on wildlife resurgence, like wolves returning, the reality is complex. Some animals may appear delicate, but long-term genetic and health impacts remain uncertain. The ecosystem's apparent recovery masks ongoing radiation effects that are difficult to quantify.

The third major published nuclear reactor meltdown,

and certainly not the last, occurred on March 11, 2011, in Fukushima, Japan. The disaster was triggered by a powerful earthquake and subsequent tsunami, which caused a backup generator to fail. Building nuclear reactors on a fault line, at low sea level, and near groundwater flowing into the ocean was ill-conceived.

The meltdown was caused by human error in design and uncontrollable natural events. These factors are impossible to mitigate fully, and the only way to prevent such disasters is to avoid nuclear power altogether. Fukushima's meltdown released radioactive materials globally. Local areas experienced high radiation levels during the incident, while lower amounts traveled across the Pacific Ocean to North America.

Precise mSv measurements for these areas vary in reports. U.S. Navy ships involved in relief efforts reported crew illnesses. The USS Ronald Reagan, with about 5,500 crew members, was among the affected vessels. Some sailors later reported health issues, including cancer and thyroid problems.

West Coast communities have seen increased cancer rates. TEPCO released treated radioactive wastewater into the Pacific, further devastating Pacific Ocean fishing industries. China and South Korea banned Japanese seafood imports due to contamination fears.

Studies show increased thyroid abnormalities in Fukushima children. The Fukushima Health Management Survey found hundreds of confirmed thyroid cancer cases among examined youth. Obtaining accurate data on thyroid cancer in Japan is difficult. Radioactive isotopes have been detected in marine life across the Pacific, raising concerns about long-term ecological consequences and food safety. Fishing grounds near Fukushima remain off-limits due to persistent contamination.

Japan faces significant problems in managing radioactive waste from the Fukushima disaster. Over 10 million one-ton plastic bags filled with contaminated soil were used in the cleanup efforts, which are expected to continue for many more decades. Due to the lack of suitable disposal sites, these bags have been distributed across approximately 100,000 locations throughout Japan, often on or adjacent to farmland.

Recent storms have further complicated the storage situation, compromising some storage sites and spreading radioactive materials. This ongoing issue highlights Japan's long-term environmental and logistical challenges in the aftermath of the Fukushima nuclear disaster.

While researching more details, I found many articles that concealed the truth. I wanted to get more information since the meltdown created beta radiation isotopes Cesium-137 and Iodine-131 that traveled through the air. Fukushima produced these isotopes during the nuclear fission process. When the reactor core melted down, these radioactive materials were released. Beta radiation doesn't penetrate the skin but can be ingested or inhaled. This radioactive material can get stuck in the throat or thyroid, causing sickness or cancer. Alpha radiation, like that from Uranium-238, 235, and 234, is gamma radiation and can travel through your body, similar to how helicopter pilots die quickly when flying over Chornobyl nuclear meltdown.

Alpha, beta, and gamma radiation differ in their penetrating power and ionizing effects on the human body. Alpha particles can be blocked by skin but are highly damaging if ingested or inhaled; beta particles can penetrate skin and cause burns, while gamma rays can pass through the entire body, causing widespread damage. These types of radiation can cause cellular damage, DNA mutations, and various health issues ranging from acute radiation sickness to long-term cancer risks, depending on the dose and exposure type.

We have several types of radiation that make us sick and cause death. Alpha, beta, and gamma radiation are already all present in nuclear reactors, submarines, ships, nuclear bombs, and medical applications. There is no completely safe zone when it comes to radiation, as even low doses can increase health risks over time.

I wanted to get actual data on thyroid cancer in Japan and found it to be complicated. According to Artificial Intelligence Perplexity (AI), it could put together some of the following information after arguing with AI. This is what AI said: In Japan's Fukushima prefecture, thyroid issues and cancers were less prevalent before the 2011 nuclear accident. Today, thyroid issues are approximately 30 to 50 times greater in the affected areas of Japan. The estimated number of thyroid cancer cases (both children and adults) in Japan after the nuclear meltdowns is an estimated 58,700.

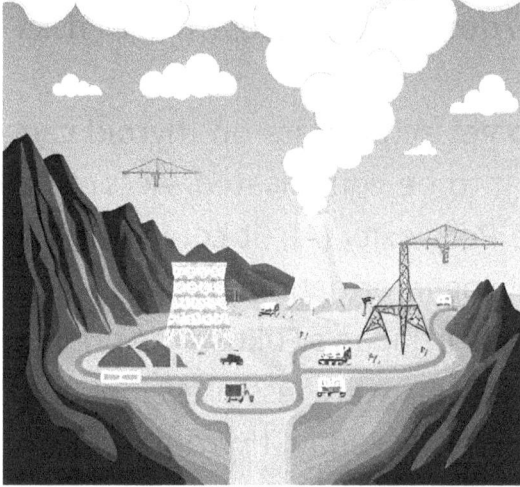

Chapter 3

Unmasking The Atom's Dark Legacy

T he nuclear fuel uranium mining initiates the nuclear fuel cycle. The Port Radium mine on Great Bear Lake in Canada's Northwest Territories was a significant source of uranium for the Manhattan Project during World War II. The local Sahtúgot'ine (Sahtu Dene) people were employed to transport and handle uranium ore without being informed of its dangers. This mining activity had long-lasting health and environmental impacts on the indigenous communities, leading to high cancer rates and the area being dubbed the "Village of Widows."

Extraction begins with open-pit or underground mining, which exposes workers to radioactive dust and radon gas. To extract uranium, ore undergoes crushing, grinding, and chemical treatment. This process generates vast quantities of unstable waste called tailings.

Tailings from nuclear mining are the waste materials left over after uranium ore has been processed to extract the uranium. These tailings typically consist of finely ground rock, water, trace metals, and residual radioactive materials, including uranium and its decay products. If not properly managed and contained, these waste byproducts pose long-term environmental and health hazards.

Conversion transforms uranium into gaseous form. Enrichment increases the concentration of fissile U-235 isotope. Fuel fabrication creates ceramic pellets, which are loaded into metal rods for reactor use. Each step produces hazardous waste.

Waste production and storage problems are significant issues with this energy source. Nuclear reactors generate high-level atomic waste in the form of spent fuel rods. These rods remain dangerous for thousands of years, and no permanent storage solution exists for this long-lived refuse.

Most spent fuel rods sit in cooling pools at reactor sites. When the pools fill, utilities move older rods to dry cask storage. Some of these casks reside in buildings constructed with simple masonry blocks, similar to retail stores made with hollow masonry blocks that can be damaged by severe weather.

The spent fuel storage at the Indian Point nuclear plant is alarmingly vulnerable. Housed in masonry block building, similar to a Kmart store, it's ill-equipped to withstand severe weather. A direct tornado hit could breach this structure, releasing radioactive material into the Hudson River nearby, contaminating the entire city of New York, killing many, and causing major health issues.

Communities nationwide have rejected proposals for permanent waste repositories. The canceled Yucca Mountain project in Nevada exemplifies public opposition to hosting nuclear refuse. Thus, atomic facility sites are de facto long-term storage facilities.

The Myth of "Clean Nuclear Energy" Nuclear power's" clean" image disregards its total environmental impact. Uranium mining scars landscapes and contaminates groundwater; mining and enrichment consume vast energy and water.

Reactor operation produces radioactive emissions and thermal pollution. Spent fuel and contaminated equipment require millennia of isolation. Decommissioning old plants leaves behind radioactive structures and radioactive soil. Nuclear accidents release long-lived radioisotopes into the environment.

Chornobyl and Fukushima demonstrated the potential for widespread, long-term contamination, rendering areas uninhabitable for generations. "Ticking Time Bomb Nuclear Plants face increasing threats from extreme weather events. Hurricanes can disrupt power supplies and cooling systems, floods may inundate critical equipment, and droughts can reduce the available cooling water.

Earthquakes pose risks of structural damage and loss of containment. Tsunamis can overwhelm seawalls and flood emergency generators. Climate instability amplifies these dangers, making plants vulnerable to unprecedented events. Aging infrastructure compounds these risks. Many U.S. reactors operate well beyond their initial design lifespans. Material degradation, outdated technology, and cumulative wear increase the likelihood of failures.

Several types of nuclear reactors, such as pressurized water power plants (PWRs), dominate the global nuclear fleet. These use high-pressure water as both coolant and moderator. Steam generators produce steam to drive turbines. Boiling Water Reactors (BWRs) allow water to cook directly in the reactor core. This more straightforward design eliminates the need for steam generators but may increase radiation exposure risks.

Other types include heavy water reactors, gas-cooled reactors, and fast neutron reactors. Each power plant presents unique safety considerations and waste management problems. Design flaws and vulnerabilities are also considered. The Three Mile Island accident revealed inadequate operator training and confusing control room design. Faulty valves and ambiguous instrument readings led to a partial meltdown.

Chornobyl's RBMK reactor lacked a containment structure. In Russian, RBMK stands for "Reaktor Bolshoy Moshchnosti Kanalnyy," which translates to "High Power Channel-type Reactor" in English. The RBMK is a Soviet-designed nuclear reactor using enriched uranium. This unique design uses graphite as its moderator and light water as coolant, a combination not found in other reactor types. It was designed for both plutonium production and electrical generation.

Its positive void coefficient made the reactor unstable at decreased power, contributing to the catastrophic explosion and fire.

A positive void coefficient in a reactor means the re-activity increases as the void content (typically steam bubbles) inside the reactor increases. This creates a po-tentially dangerous positive feedback loop. In the RBMK reactor design used at Chornobyl, this characteristic was a fundamental design flaw that made the reactor unstable and prone to sudden power surges, especially at low power levels, contributing significantly to the dis-aster.

Fukushima Daiichi's seawall was under designed to withstand the tsunami. Basement emergency genera-tors flooded, causing a loss of power and cooling. Hy-drogen explosions breached secondary containment, releasing radiation.

The Nuclear Regulatory Commission has extended op-erating licenses for most U.S. reactors by 20 years or more, pushing many plants well beyond their 40-year design lives. The embrittlement of reactor vessels raises concerns about catastrophic failure. Degraded piping systems may leak radioactive water, and outdated ana-log control systems lack modern safety features.

Deferred maintenance due to economic pressures further compromises safety margins. Staff reductions and budget cuts affect inspection and repair schedules. These factors combine to elevate the risk of significant time accidents.

During the Cold War, government-sponsored scientists appeared on television to promote atomic power. These experts assured viewers of its safety, glossing over risks and uncertainties. This propaganda campaign sought to allay public fears and garner support for nuclear expansion.

The Manhattan Project exposed numerous scientists and workers to radiation hazards. Enrico Fermi's team conducted early reactor experiments with minimal shielding.

Enrico Fermi, an Italian-born physicist, was a key player in the Manhattan Project. He developed the first nuclear reactor (Chicago Pile-1) and contributed to the creation of the atomic bomb. He worked in many areas, including Chicago, Los Alamos, Hanford, and Oak Ridge. He played important roles in reactor design and plutonium production and witnessed the Trinity test before becoming a professor at the University of Chicago.

The Trinity test, conducted on July 16, 1945, at 5:29 a.m. in the Jornada del Muerto desert near Socorro, New

Mexico, was the world's first nuclear explosion and the only test before the atomic bombings of Japan. This event, which detonated a plutonium implosion device nicknamed "The Gadget" with a yield of 18.6 kilotons, marked the beginning of the Atomic Age. Just three weeks later, atomic weapons were used on Hiroshima and Nagasaki on August 6 and 9, respectively. The test's success validated the design later used in the Fat Man bomb dropped on Nagasaki.

However, the Trinity test had lasting health consequences for nearby residents, with studies suggesting increased cancer rates in the surrounding counties. The Centers for Disease Control found that locals were exposed to radiation levels 10,000 times higher than currently allowed, and the National Cancer Institute estimated several hundred excess cancer cases over 75 years, primarily thyroid cancer, due to the test.

Plutonium processing at Hanford released radioactive iodine into the environment. Many project participants later developed cancers and other radiation-induced illnesses. The actual toll remains unknown due to secrecy and inadequate record-keeping. These early atomic pioneers paid a heavy price for their groundbreaking work.

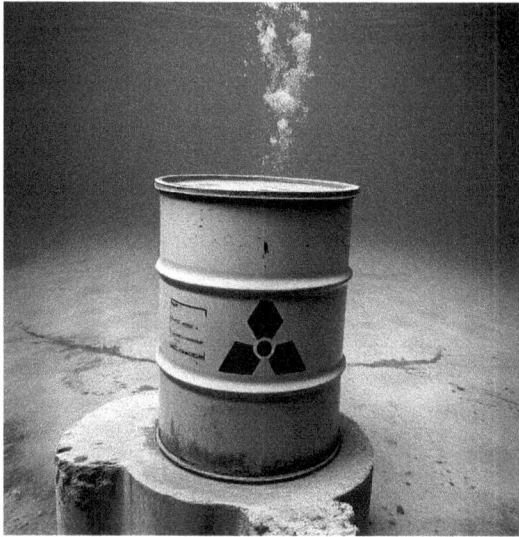

Chapter 4

The Global Graveyard Of Atomic Waste

We discussed some nuclear contaminations or accidents in previous chapters and will continue to do so in future chapters. Every location where radiation or nuclear activity stops, whether due to an accident, a dump, a storage facility, or other causes, becomes a new graveyard of atomic waste. Let's look at some of these graveyards that destroy our planet.

In 1957, the Kyshtym disaster at the Mayak facility in Chelyabinsk Oblast, Soviet Union, released 20 MCi (megacuries) of radioactivity. This release was equivalent to 20 million curies or approximately 7.4×10^{17} becquerels, where one megacurie equals one million curies (with one curie being 3.7×10^{10} becquerels). This event contaminated 20,000 square kilometers, the size of West Virginia, with cesium-137 and strontium-90, which have half-lives of about 30 years. The area remains hazardous, with groundwater pollution extending to the Arctic Ocean.

Germany, the world's first rocket inventor, uses multiple sites to deal with nuclear waste storage. Germany has had no active nuclear power plants since April 15, 2023, when it shut down its last three operational reactors: Isar 2, Emsland, and Neckarwestheim 2. This marked the end of Germany's planned nuclear exit, which began after the 2011 Fukushima disaster. The country phased out all 17 of its nuclear reactors over more than a decade and is now decommissioning 31 reactors.

Germany has shifted focus to renewable energy sources as part of its Energiewende policy. Despite some calls to reconsider nuclear power due to energy security concerns, there are no plans to restart or build new nuclear plants in Germany. The country has no single sizeable atomic dump. It uses numerous sites for various types of nuclear waste. Each site presents its problems. These unique problems include but are not limited to, aging CASTOR containers nearing their design lifespan, water ingress issues at the Asse II mine, a lack of a permanent solution for high-level waste, and public opposition to waste transportation and storage sites.

About 1,200 CASTOR containers—Cask for Storage and Transport of Radioactive Material — are stored at 17 interim sites across Germany. These containers hold spent fuel rods from nuclear power plants, including Biblis, Brokdorf, Grohnde, and Gundremmingen. The number will increase to 1,800 containers.

Schacht Konrad, a former iron ore mine near Salzgitter, will store low and medium-level nuclear waste. Low and medium-level waste includes contaminated equipment, clothing, and materials from atomic plant operations, containing isotopes such as cobalt-60, cesium-137, and strontium-90. It will hold 303,000 cubic meters of waste, equivalent to about 39,629 10-yard dump trucks. The site is under construction. Operations begin in the early 2030s.

The Asse II mine contains 125,787 low-level drums and 1,293 medium-level waste containers from nuclear power plants, research facilities, and hospitals. Due to instability in the salt structure and cracks in the rock, it faces water leakage and instability issues. Water ingress threatens to spread contamination, which is currently contained but remains a risk. Inadequate records obscure the full extent of stored isotopes.

The Gorleben site was eliminated in 2020 due to geological concerns, including issues with the salt dome's stability and potential groundwater contamination. Germany will eventually select a site for permanently storing high-level radioactive waste, including spent fuel rods and reprocessing residues.

The process, expected to finish in the 2040s, is regulated by the Site Selection Act (StandAG) and comprises three phases: identifying sub-areas and siting regions for surface exploration, surface exploration of selected areas and proposal of suitable sites for underground exploration, and proposal of possible repository sites. It started with a "white map" approach, considering all of Germany, and has identified 90 sub-areas covering about 54% of Germany's onshore area.

The process involves extensive public participation and is overseen by the Federal Company for Radioactive Waste Disposal (BGE) and the Federal Office for Safety of Nuclear Waste Management (BASE). Construction is expected to start in the 2060s, with estimated costs in the tens of billions of dollars. Given the complexity of the process and the extended timeframe, it seems they have no clear idea of how this will ultimately unfold.

Hanford in Washington State, USA, holds 56 million gallons of waste from plutonium production. Leaks have occurred in underground tanks. Workers report health issues from toxic vapors. Contamination risks to the Columbia River persist. The site contains long-lived isotopes like plutonium-239, with a half-life of 24,100 years. The Columbia River, which flows for nearly 1,250 miles through the Pacific Northwest, has been directly impacted by Hanford's operations.

Past practices allowed contaminated water to be returned to the river without treatment until 1972. Studies show that radioactive materials from Hanford have reached the Pacific Ocean 200 miles away, affecting fish and drinking water. During the Cold War, Hanford originally produced plutonium for over 60,000 nuclear weapons. The site spans 586 square miles, equivalent to half the size of Rhode Island.

Underground tunnels contain train cars full of nuclear waste, with one tunnel collapsing in 2017. Several decommissioned nuclear submarines await dismantling at the site. The total waste volume at Hanford is estimated at 1.7 trillion gallons, including liquid waste, contaminated soil, and groundwater. To date, cleanup costs have exceeded $170 billion, with estimates for total cleanup ranging to $640 billion. The site has a history of accidents, including the 1949 "Green Run" intentional release of radioactive iodine-131.

The "Green Run" was a secret U.S. Government experiment conducted on December 2-3, 1949, at the Hanford Site plutonium production facility in Eastern Washington. It involved the intentional release of radioactive fission products, primarily iodine-131 and xenon-133, into the atmosphere. The experiment aimed to test methods for detecting Soviet nuclear weapons production by tracking and measuring the spread of airborne radioactive material. The Green Run released 8,000 to 12,000 curies of iodine-131, significantly more than the 15 curies released during the Three Mile Island accident. This deliberate release showered nearby communities with radiation and resulted in long-term health problems for many "Downwinders," including increased cancer rates and lymphatic illnesses.

Yucca Mountain, located in Nevada, was designated by Congress in 1987 as the sole site for a national deep geological repository for high-level nuclear waste and spent nuclear fuel. From the outset, the project encountered significant problems and opposition; the site selection was criticized as politically motivated rather than scientifically based, with Nevada officials and residents strongly opposing the idea. After all, who would want a radioactive site in their backyard? Concerns about the site's geology were raised, particularly regarding potential water infiltration and seismic activity—why would anyone consider placing a radioactive facility on a fault line?

Transportation risks associated with moving nuclear waste across the country to Yucca Mountain were also significant issues. These were compounded by the repository's planned capacity of 70,000 metric tons, which was deemed insufficient for all existing and projected nuclear waste. Remember those new freeway signs nationwide indicating which roads were acceptable for transporting this hazardous material? The taxpayers paid for that, too.

"No Hazardous Materials" or "No HM" signs on certain freeways and roads prohibiting the transport of dangerous cargo, including spent nuclear fuel rods. These restrictions, implemented to protect public safety and the environment, are part of a complex regulatory framework developed by the U.S. Department of Transportation (DOT) and the Nuclear Regulatory Commission (NRC). While carriers of highway route-controlled quantity shipments, such as spent nuclear fuel, are required to use "preferred routing" and prepare detailed written plans, there's a critical oversight: the towns, cities, rivers, and forests these hazardous materials routes pass through never got to vote on these designations. Consequently, a non-knowing village would not be prepared if an accident occurred.

Nevada officials and residents have opposed the project for years, arguing that the site is geologically unsuitable and poses significant risks. Currently, over 85,000 metric tons of spent nuclear fuel and high-level radioactive waste remain stored in temporary facilities at more than 100 reactor sites across the country.

In 2010, the Obama administration moved to terminate the Yucca Mountain project by filing a motion to withdraw its license application with the Nuclear Regulatory Commission and cutting funding, halting further development. This decision was met with legal fights from several states and organizations. As it stands now, the Yucca Mountain project remains in limbo—neither fully terminated nor actively pursued. Over three decades, the Yucca Mountain nuclear waste repository project has cost American taxpayers nearly $15 billion, yet no nuclear waste has been stored at the site.

Despite electricity consumers contributing over $56 billion to the Nuclear Waste Fund, the federal government's failure to take ownership of nuclear waste has led to $6.9 billion in utility payments for on-site storage costs, with potential liabilities reaching up to $50 billion. Ultimately, taxpayers bear the financial burden of this stalled project, paying approximately $2.2 million daily due to the government's inability to fulfill its legal obligation to manage nuclear waste. So, while Yucca Mountain was intended to be a solution for nuclear waste disposal, it has become a costly burden for taxpayers who never voted on this issue.

France's La Hague reprocessing plant, located on the Cotentin Peninsula, has operated since 1976. It features three large storage pools to hold spent nuclear fuel before processing. While no significant leaks have been reported, concerns persist about the plant's environmental impact and role as a dumping ground for radioactive waste. Greenpeace alleges that La Hague discharges 270,000 gallons of liquid radioactive waste daily into the English Channel as Greenpeace alleges. Studies have detected radioactive contamination in marine organisms such as fish, crabs, and seaweed. Long-lived isotopes like iodine-129 bioaccumulate in the food chain, potentially impacting larger marine animals and humans consuming seafood from the area.

While no direct evidence links the plant to mass die-offs of fish or marine mammals, radioactive materials from La Hague have spread across the North Sea and even into Arctic waters. Cancer rates are reportedly higher in the region surrounding the plant, though a direct causal link remains unproven. The discharges have also raised concerns about fisheries, as public perception of contamination can harm demand even when pollution levels are below harmful limits. Overall, La Hague's operations highlight serious risks to marine ecosystems and human health, warranting further research and stricter oversight.

The La Hague nuclear reprocessing plant in France processes approximately 1,100 metric tons of used nuclear fuel annually, extracting reusable materials like plutonium for MOX fuel production. MOX fuel, or mixed oxide fuel, is a blend of plutonium and depleted uranium, typically containing 3% to 10% plutonium. This fuel allows for plutonium recycling from spent nuclear fuel and weapons, although only a fraction is recycled at La Hague.

During reprocessing, isotopes such as iodine-129 (with a half-life of 15.7 million years) and strontium-90 (with a half-life of 29 years) are released. Critics argue that the recycling of nuclear materials at La Hague is often exaggerated, suggesting that the facility functions more as a taxpayer-funded waste storage site than an efficient recycling facility. The ongoing storage of high-level waste at La Hague contributes to environmental degradation and poses long-term risks to public health.

As La Hague continues accumulating nuclear waste without a permanent disposal solution, it highlights the persistent challenges surrounding atomic waste management in France. The facility's operations raise concerns about the effectiveness of nuclear fuel recycling and the long-term environmental and health impacts of storing radioactive materials with such extended half-lives.

Great Britain's land is dotted with defunct MOX nuclear power plants and massive concrete structures that have become radioactive relics of a bygone era. These facilities, designed to recycle plutonium and uranium from spent nuclear fuel, were initially built to manage atomic waste and reduce dependence on fresh uranium. However, many of these plants had short operational lives, resulting in significant environmental mishaps. Now standing as some of the largest "gravestones" known to mankind, these decommissioned plants are often located near national landmarks, relics, and parks. Some examples include the Sellafield MOX Plant in Cumbria, the Dungeness A plant in Kent, Bradwell (closed in 2002), and Berkeley (ceased operations in 1989). Despite no longer functioning, these structures will remain radioactive for centuries.

The decommissioning process for these MOX plants in Great Britain is a long-term endeavor defining the complexities of nuclear facility closure. The Sellafield site encompasses multiple facilities and is not expected to be fully decommissioned until 2120. The Calder Hall plant has a phased decommissioning plan: refueling and removing most buildings by 2032, followed by a care and maintenance phase until 2104, with final demolition and site clearance scheduled from 2105 to 2114. This extended timeline, spanning 90 years, raises questions about long-term planning and responsibility.

That is 90 years. Who plans this far into the future? That's after four more generations. So my kids' kids' kids will be the ones to clean this up." This long-term commitment to managing nuclear waste and decommissioning facilities shows the complex and lasting impact of atomic energy decisions made decades ago, leaving a significant burden for future generations to bear.

The Dungeness A plant was decommissioned in 2006, but full site clearance will take several decades, and no specific date has been set for its complete removal. Similarly, the Bradwell plant, closed in 2002, has no definitive timeline for its total dismantling. The Berkeley plant ceased operations in 1989, yet its complete removal will continue without a precise end date.

Despite being non-operational, these facilities remain radioactive for many years due to the residual materials housed within them. The isotopes present can have half-lives extending into thousands of years, necessitating long-term monitoring and maintenance. For instance, plutonium-239 has a half-life of 24,100 years, which will continue to pose risks long after the plants are decommissioned. If a generation lasts 25 years, it takes 25,000 for a half-life of 1,000 generations.

Complete removal plans for these sites have not been finalized, with estimates suggesting that some may take hundreds of years to remediate fully. This raises critical questions about the decision to build such massive concrete structures without comprehensive plans for their eventual dismantling. Ultimately, maintaining and monitoring these radioactive monuments for centuries poses ongoing challenges for future generations and highlights the need for better planning in nuclear energy management.

The Farallon Islands dump off San Francisco contains 47,800 waste containers across 1,400 square kilometers of seafloor. It was dumped between 1946 and 1970, and many drums have deteriorated and are leaking. The site is now a marine sanctuary, and isotopes present include plutonium-239 (half-life of 24,100 years) and americium-241 (432 years). This dumping was legal under the authority of the Atomic Energy

Commission, but the long-term environmental impacts remain a concern.

New York's Atlantic coast dump site, located 120 miles offshore, received thousands of waste drums from 1946 to 1962. The exact number and condition of the containers are unknown, but leakage threatens marine life and coastal communities. Long-lived isotopes like plutonium may persist for millennia, impacting local ecosystems. This site is not actively monitored and continues to create havoc on surrounding waters and wildlife.

The Kara Sea dump in Russia contains 17 nuclear reactors and 19,000 waste containers, remnants of Soviet-era disposal practices. These practices have left a legacy of pollution in the Arctic Ocean, with isotopes like cesium-137 (half-life of 30 years) and strontium-90 (29 years) contaminating the marine environment. Melting sea ice may expose more waste, which will continue to cause havoc on local wildlife and human populations.

The West Lake Landfill in St. Louis, Missouri, contains uranium processing waste from the 1970s. An underground fire has been burning since 2010, threatening to spread contamination. Radium-226 (half-life of 1,600 years) poses long-term risks to groundwater and nearby communities. This radioactive waste was illegally dumped, causing residents ongoing environmental and health hazards.

Sellafield in Cumbria, England, discharges radioactive waste into the Irish Sea while reprocessing nuclear fuel. The site has shown elevated radioactivity levels in marine life due to isotopes like technetium-99 (half-life of 211,000 years). This facility is actively monitored but continues to raise concerns about its impact on local ecosystems. Elevated levels of radioactivity have been detected in seaweed and shellfish.

India's Jadugoda uranium mine in Jharkhand produces tailings containing radioactive waste. Dams holding this material risk failure, potentially contaminating local water sources. Local populations report increased cancer rates and congenital disabilities linked to exposure. Radon gas, a decay product of uranium, contaminates the air and soil around the mine.

Beyond the well-documented cases, countries like Ukraine, Russia, Great Britain, and Germany deal with all problems of nuclear waste disposal. The Netherlands, too, confronts the complex task of managing radioactive materials that threaten local ecosystems. These atomic waste repositories house hazardous substances with half-lives spanning centuries or millennia, presenting an enduring risk to the environment and future generations.

The global landscape of nuclear waste management continues to evolve, with new disposal sites being evaluated and selected worldwide. After a meticulous 14-year process, Canada has approved a nuclear waste disposal site, with the Nuclear Waste Management Organization (NWMO) selecting Wabigoon Lake Ojibway Nation and the Ignace area in northern Ontario as potential hosts. This decision marks a significant step in addressing the long-term storage of radioactive materials, but it also raises important questions about community involvement and safety.

The selection process has been controversial, with the NWMO offering substantial financial incentives to small communities willing to host the repository. Critics argue that these payments, often amounting to millions of dollars, unduly influence municipal decision-making. While the NWMO maintains that these funds are for conducting studies, some view the arrangement as a form of coercion, likening it to a horse accepting a carrot. The voting process, which allows municipalities rather than individual residents to make the final decision, has further fueled concerns about the true nature of community consent.

The transportation of nuclear waste has raised significant concerns, particularly regarding safety on accident-prone Highways 11 and 17. The plan to ship radioactive materials daily for nine months each year has alarmed residents along these routes, who face potential risks without having a say. Special teams would be needed to handle emergencies, and once a town agrees to host a waste site, they cannot change their decision, adding to the situation's complexity.

The proximity of transportation routes to the Great Lakes and major rivers poses substantial risks to critical water resources. An accident could lead to radioactive materials contaminating vital freshwater systems, potentially affecting drinking water sources for millions of people. Given the long half-lives of many radioactive isotopes, the long-lasting impact of such an event is particularly worrisome.

Residents, officials, and lawmakers have voiced serious concerns about these risks. For example, in Belleville, Michigan, the city manager highlighted the threat to Belleville Lake, part of the Huron River system flowing into Lake Erie. Senators have opposed proposals to ship radioactive steam generators through the Great Lakes and St. Lawrence Seaway, fearing it could set a dangerous precedent for transporting high-level radioactive materials.

Environmental groups and local communities have raised alarms about long-term risks. Stop the Great Lakes Nuclear Dump estimates that a leak from a proposed deep geological repository near Lake Huron could impact 40 million people in Canada and the United States. The possibility of radionuclides entering the lake, even thousands of years later, remains a significant concern.

These sites mentioned above represent a fraction of global nuclear waste dumps. What constitutes an international nuclear waste dump? Is it small or large, and does it leak or pollute? These areas will be contaminated for many generations, with some lasting 1,000 generations if you count one generation as 25 years. The full extent of environmental and health impacts remains unknown; however, people are getting sick and dying everywhere around the world every day.

Humanity's atomic ambitions have created an enduring toxic inheritance. Fishermen continue to catch and consume radioactive fish, while unexplained die-offs of fish, animals, and birds occur globally. The media shows us images of skinny, starving polar bears. Are these polar bears dying from starvation, or are they emaciated due to leukemia caused by radioactive contamination of the Arctic Sea?

MARKO VOVK

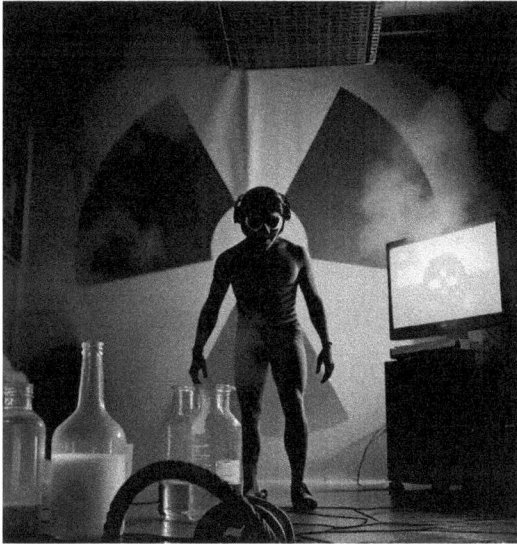

Chapter 5

Nuclear Human Experiments

During the Cold War, the U.S. government conducts secret radiation experiments on unsuspecting citizens. The goal is to study radiation effects on humans and develop protective measures for nuclear warfare. These experiments often target vulnerable populations in hospitals, prisons, and institutions.

At Vanderbilt University, from 1945 to 1949, over 800 pregnant women receive radioactive iron without consent. Seven children die from cancer before age 10, and at least 42 develop various forms of cancer. Some families file lawsuits, resulting in settlements for some affected families.

Researchers at the University of Rochester injected plutonium into 18 patients between 1945 and 1947. The experiments aim to study plutonium's effects on human health without patients' informed consent. Dr. Stafford Warren leads the study as part of the classified Manhattan Project.

Ebb Cade, a 53-year-old African American worker, enters the hospital with broken bones from a car accident. Doctors inject him with 4.7 micrograms of plutonium without his knowledge. Cade experiences tooth loss, and his bone fractures never fully heal.

Albert Stevens, admitted for suspected stomach cancer, receives a plutonium injection. Doctors later discover he doesn't have cancer but doesn't inform him of the infusion. Stevens lives for 20 years, unknowingly carrying high plutonium levels in his body. A 4-year-old boy with bone cancer receives a plutonium injection at Strong Memorial Hospital. His parents are told it's an "experimental treatment" without mentioning plutonium. The boy dies 8 months later from his cancer.

In Washington and Oregon prisons (1963-1973), doctors conduct testicular irradiation experiments on 131 prisoners. They study radiation effects on sperm production and testicular function. Some prisoners report sterility and increased cancer risk later in life. Detailed long-term health impacts remain undocumented due to limited follow-up studies, which are typical for this entire industry.

Researchers at San Quentin Prison, California, expose prisoners to whole-body radiation to study blood formation and immune response. The experiments aim to understand radiation's effects on the human body. However, available sources do not document long-term health consequences for these prisoners.

At Fernald State School (1946-1953), researchers feed radioactive iron and calcium to 74 developmentally disabled children in oatmeal. They aim to study nutrient absorption. The experiments became public in 1993, leading to a class-action lawsuit and a $1.85 million settlement. Long-term health effects on the children remain unclear.

At Willowbrook State School (1950s-1970s), researchers deliberately infect mentally disabled children with hepatitis and then conduct radiation experiments. They aim to track disease progression and test treatments.

The unethical nature of these experiments led to public outrage when exposed in the 1970s. Long-term health impacts on children are not well-documented in available sources.

Let's go back and back to Germany and see what the Nazi regime did using radiation and radioactive isotopes on human subjects. The horrific experiments conducted during World War II reveal a dark chapter in medical history, where ethical boundaries were disregarded in the pursuit of scientific knowledge. From high-altitude simulations to sterilization procedures, these experiments inflicted unimaginable suffering on countless victims.

High-Altitude Experiments (Dachau, 1942): Dr. Sigmund Rascher conducted these experiments on approximately 200 prisoners to study the physiological effects of high altitudes. The prisoners were placed in low-pressure chambers to simulate conditions at altitudes up to 68,000 feet. Many subjects suffered severe health consequences, with 80 dying from exposure. The long-term outcomes for survivors included various health issues related to the extreme conditions.

Freezing Experiments (Dachau, 1942): While these experiments primarily focused on the effects of extreme cold, they often involved combinations of physical stressors, including radiation exposure. Prisoners were subjected to ice water immersion or left naked in freezing temperatures for hours. Many victims died from exposure or suffered permanent disabilities. The overall stress from these experiments could have compounded any radiation effects experienced during other Nazi medical studies.

Radiation Exposure for Cancer Studies (Auschwitz, 1940s): Some prisoners were exposed to high levels of radiation under the guise of treatment for cancer. Specific numbers of affected individuals are not well-documented, but many developed acute radiation syndrome and suffered long-lasting health effects. The outcomes included increased cancer rates among survivors and premature deaths linked to radiation exposure.

X-Ray Radiation on Children (Auschwitz, 1940s): Children at Auschwitz were subjected to X-ray radiation without consent or knowledge of the risks. The exact numbers are unclear, but many suffered from radiation burns and long-term health complications such as cancer and developmental issues. The outcomes for these children often included severe congenital disabilities or early death.

Plutonium Injection Experiments (Various Camps, 1940s): Some prisoners received injections of plutonium to study its effects on human health. The exact numbers of those injected vary, but many developed severe health issues such as organ failure and cancer. Outcomes often included premature death due to the toxicity of plutonium.

Bone Marrow Experiments (Auschwitz, 1940s): Researchers exposed prisoners to radiation to study its effects on bone marrow and blood production. Specific numbers are not well-documented, but victims frequently suffer from anemia and other blood disorders as a result of radiation exposure. Long-term outcomes included chronic health issues and increased mortality rates among survivors.

Radiation Experiments on Pregnant Women (Auschwitz, 1940s): Pregnant women were subjected to X-ray radiation without consent to study fetal development under radiation exposure. Many women were Jewish prisoners or other marginalized groups. The exact numbers are unclear, but many children suffered severe congenital disabilities or died shortly after birth due to the exposure.

Infection with Radioactive Materials (Various Camps, 1940s): Prisoners were deliberately infected with radioactive materials to study disease progression and treatment responses. Specific details about who was infected vary by camp, but many experienced severe health complications and premature deaths due to the experiments. Long-term outcomes included chronic illnesses and increased mortality rates among survivors.

Human Experimentation for Medical Research (Various Camps, 1940s): Various camps conducted experiments on unwilling subjects to gather data on human responses to radiation exposure. The exact number of victims is complex to determine, but these experiments resulted in countless deaths and lifelong suffering for survivors. Many individuals faced severe health complications due to their exposure during these unethical studies.

Following the atomic bombings of Hiroshima and Nagasaki, approximately 120,000 survivors are monitored to understand the long-term effects of this isotope contact. Many develop leukemia and other cancers over the decades, with a significant portion of issues going unreported due to stigma and lack of comprehensive studies. Despite knowing the dangers of these energy sources almost 80 years ago, authorities continue implementing harmful practices that affect countless lives.

In the UK, researchers expose thousands of patients to unnecessary X-rays while studying tuberculosis treatments. This leads to increased cancer rates among those treated, with long-term studies revealing significant impacts, including a rise in breast malignancy cases affecting thousands. This issue extends beyond the USA to countries like Canada and the UK, where women employed to paint watch dials with radium-based paint ingest radioactive material through lip-pointing their brushes. Many develop severe health issues such as bone cancer and anemia, resulting in numerous lawsuits filed against employers for negligence, with hundreds affected by these practices.

Atomic Energy of Canada Limited conducts experiments on hospital patients involving radiation exposure to study radioactive isotopes in cancer care. Patients receive injections without full consent, leading to severe complications and increased cancer risk. Approximately 600,000 workers exposed to high levels of contact during cleanup efforts after the Chornobyl disaster developed acute radiation syndrome and long-term health issues such as thyroid malignancy. Today, estimates suggest that only around 200,000 of these workers remain alive and healthy, with many suffering from chronic illnesses linked to their exposure.

After a nuclear accident in the Soviet Union, thousands of residents in the Chelyabinsk region are exposed to radioactive fallout. Many suffer from radiation sickness and long-term health problems, including increased cancer rates, with limited governmental information provided. Residents of the Marshall Islands are exposed to atomic bombs from U.S. nuclear tests conducted in the area, leading to severe issues like thyroid tumors and other illnesses related to exposure.

Compensation claims are ongoing for affected individuals due to the long-term consequences of these tests. Aboriginal miners in Australia face significant exposure in uranium mines without proper safety measures or health monitoring. Many develop lung cancer and other respiratory illnesses due to prolonged engagement with radioactive dust, with limited recognition or compensation for their suffering.

The Soviet government conducts experiments on prisoners and people with a mental health condition involving exposure to study its effects on humans. Many subjects suffer from severe health complications, including cancers and organ damage, with little follow-up care provided after these unethical experiments. During nuclear testing across various countries like Algeria, local populations are exposed to radiation from atmospheric tests without adequate warnings or protections. Many residents report long-term issues, including cancers and genetic disorders among subsequent generations.

These experiments mentioned above show a global pattern of unethical human experimentation involving radiation interaction, resulting in profound suffering and lasting consequences for countless victims involved in these studies. Despite historical lessons learned from these tragedies, humanity continues to repeat its mistakes, often prioritizing scientific advancement over ethical considerations and human rights.

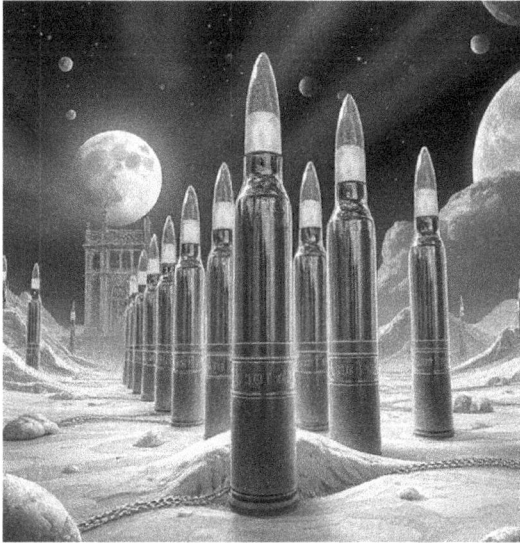

Chapter 6

Nuclear Arsenal

G ermany developed and deployed the first operational attack missiles during World War II. The V-1 flying bomb, launched on June 13, 1944, became the world's first cruise missile. Germany launched approximately 10,000 V-1s at targets in Britain and 9,000 at Continental Europe. The V-2 rocket, launched on September 8, 1944, became the world's first ballistic missile.

Germany launches 3,172 V-2 rockets against Allied cities like London, Paris, and Antwerp. These German "Vengeance Weapons" represent a major technological breakthrough in missile technology. A pulsejet engine powers the V-1 and launches from ground sites or aircraft. The V-2 is a liquid-fueled rocket that reaches supersonic speeds. These weapons strike large targets like cities. They cause significant casualties and damage, killing around 6,200 British civilians with V-1 attacks. V-2 attacks kill over 7,000 people.

IG Farben, a German chemical conglomerate, rents Jewish people from Hitler to make these bombs. Wernher von Braun directs the operation, paying workers $1 per day. People are brought to a secret mountain facility where they make the missiles. Only missiles and body bags leave the mountain.

After the war, these scientists left Germany and worked for the USA and Russia under classified programs like Project Paperclip, which jump-started their missile and space programs. Soon after, the military-industrial complex became a reality. IG Farben became part of companies like BASF (Baden Aniline and Soda Factory), Bayer, and Hoechst. This technology and nuclear advancements form the world's future nuclear arsenal.

The first nuclear device ever detonated was the "Gadget" during the Trinity test on July 16, 1945, in New Mexico. This plutonium implosion-type bomb was a prototype for the Fat Man bomb, later used in Nagasaki. The test produced a mushroom cloud that rose to over 38,000 feet. Despite assurances of safety, the Trinity test posed significant radiation hazards. The radioactive cloud dispersed toward the north-northeast, dropping fallout over a wide area.

Several ranch families received significant radiation exposure in the following weeks. The government downplayed these risks at the time. In total, the United States conducted over 1,000 nuclear tests between 1945 and 1992. This included over 200 atmospheric tests, over 800 underground tests, and several high-altitude and space tests. The fallout from these tests contaminated thousands of square miles of land and water. Common radioactive isotopes produced included strontium-90 (half-life of 29 years) and cesium-137 (half-life of 30 years). We now know these tests were not safe, as many people exposed to fallout later developed cancers and other health issues.

On August 6, 1945, the United States dropped the "Little Boy" atomic bomb on Hiroshima, Japan. This uranium gun-type bomb was developed at Los Alamos Laboratory under J. Robert Oppenheimer. A separate plutonium bomb was produced at Hanford, Washington. The Hiroshima bombing killed an estimated 147,000 people, including thousands of children who were outside clearing firebreaks. Many victims were instantly vaporized, leaving only shadows burned into surfaces. Survivors suffered horrific burns and radiation sickness. Thousands more died of cancers and other effects in subsequent years.

On August 9, 1945, the United States dropped the "Fat Man" plutonium implosion bomb on Nagasaki. This killed an estimated 74,000 people initially. Survivors described people with melted eyes and skin sloughing off their bodies. The bombings led to Japan's surrender, ending World War II. Some historians argue Japan was already trying to surrender before the atomic bombings. Still, the US proceeded anyway after investing so much in developing the bombs during the secret Manhattan Project. However, this remains debated.

In 1954, the US tested its first deliverable hydrogen bomb, Castle Bravo, at Bikini Atoll. This 15-megaton blast was 1,000 times more potent than the Hiroshima bomb. It was developed to create a weapon capable of destroying entire cities. The test contaminated nearby islands and a Japanese fishing boat 100 miles away. Crew members suffered radiation sickness, with many dying later. Parts of the Marshall Islands remain contaminated today, with restricted access. Marine life in the area continues to show elevated radiation levels 70 years later.

Nuclear warheads are everywhere, waiting to be used. Several types are categorized as deployed, reserved, or retired. Deployed warheads are installed on ICBMs (Intercontinental Ballistic Missiles), SLBMs (Submarine-Launched Ballistic Missiles), or strategic bombers, while reserve warheads are stored for potential activation.

Approximately 13,000 retired warheads await dismantlement, stored separately yet still radioactive. Globally, 14,000 nuclear warheads exist: 3,700 deployed, 5,000 reserved, 400 plus underground, and 3,900 retired. Unknown numbers are sunk with ships and submarines underwater.

The USA possesses 5,044 nuclear warheads: 1,770 deployed, 1,938 reserved, and 1,336 retired, with 400 in underground silos. Russia has 5,977 warheads: 1,710 deployed, 2,670 stored, and 1,200 retired. China maintains 500 warheads, with 24 deployed and 476 stored. These weapons contribute to an ongoing nuclear extinction event, raising questions about their purpose: protection or control through fear and division.

Seven other countries possess atomic weapons. France holds 290 warheads (280 deployed, ten stored), the United Kingdom has 225 (120 deployed, 105 stored), Pakistan and India each have around 170 stored, Israel keeps 90 stored, and North Korea retains 50 stored. Exact numbers remain uncertain due to classified programs, leaving the true extent of global nuclear arsenals unknown.

These arsenal weapons also have many accidents because they happen, and many are inevitable. On August 5, 1950, in California, a B-29 bomber crashed, causing a nuclear bomb's high explosive to detonate, killing 19 people. At Kirtland AFB, New Mexico, on May 22, 1957, a B-36 dropped a Mark 17 thermonuclear weapon, which was destroyed by its high explosive material. On October 11, 1957, at Homestead Air Force Base, Florida, a B-47 crashed during takeoff, causing a nuclear bomb to burn in the resulting fire. A B-47 carrying a sealed-pit nuclear weapon crashed during a simulated takeoff at Sidi Slimane Air Base, Morocco, on January 31, 1958, causing some contamination.

Additional incidents involving bombs occurred worldwide. At Greenham Common US Base, England, on February 28, 1958, a B-47E jettisoned fuel tanks, one of which hit a hangar near a parked B-47E carrying a 1.1 megaton B28 nuclear bomb. On March 11, 1958, in Florence, South Carolina, a B-47E accidentally dropped an unarmed atomic weapon, which exploded on impact, causing property damage and injuries. A B-52 broke up in mid-air over Goldsboro, North Carolina, on January 24, 1961, dropping two nuclear bombs, with one coming close to detonating. On January 17, 1966, in Palomares, Spain, a B-52 collided with a refueling tanker, dropping four hydrogen bombs, two of which released radioactive material upon impact. Each of these bizarre events has stories. Let's look at the Palomares Spain Plane collision,

On January 17, 1966, a B-52G bomber collided with a KC-135 tanker over Palomares, Spain, at 31,000 feet, killing seven crew members. Four Mark 28 thermonuclear bombs fall from the B-52. One bomb lands intact on land. Two detonate conventionally on impact, spreading plutonium contamination—the fourth plunges into the sea. The deep-sea submersible Alvin aids in the fourth bomb's recovery during Project Alpha, which takes 80 days to complete.

Operation Moist Mop begins, involving 1,700 US servicemen. They remove 1,500 tons of contaminated soil and ship it to the Savannah River Site in South Carolina. The operation costs $80 million. US officials initially lied to the public, claiming no nuclear contamination or threat despite this being the world's most significant plutonium leak accident at the time. Secretary of Defense McNamara and President Johnson receive briefings. The incident strains U.S.-S.-Spain relations.

In 2004, a second cleanup removed 211,888 cubic feet of soil, costing $32 million. In 2015, the US agreed to remove 1,765,733 cubic feet more. Villagers collect radioactive souvenirs, unaware of the danger. The area is fenced, yet rabbit hunters continue their activities despite contamination.

Approximately 38 years later, land and people undergo testing. Some cleanup workers and residents report illnesses consistent with radiation exposure, including various cancers, respiratory problems, and skin conditions. However, establishing a direct link between these health issues and the incident proves difficult due to limited long-term health studies and the passage of time. Health concerns persist for workers and residents, and monitoring continues. The incident remains secretive initially, with limited public disclosure.

On January 21, 1968, a B-52 bomber carrying four thermonuclear weapons crashed onto the sea ice near Thule Air Base in Greenland after the crew ejected due to an onboard fire. These weapons of mass destruction had explosives in the arsenal detonated upon impact, dispersing radioactive material across the ice. While parts of three bombs were definitively identified during the cleanup operation codenamed "Project Crested Ice," the fate of one bomb remains uncertain. Despite an extensive three-year search effort, including the use of submarines, one bomb component - a secondary stage cylinder containing uranium and lithium deuteride - was never recovered and is believed to have sunk through the ice to the seafloor. If you can believe this, we have a lost nuclear bomb under Greenland somewhere, and it's still radio silence.

Russia and the United States control 88% of the world's nuclear weapons, with 3,904 warheads deployed and about 2,100 on high alert. NATO's nuclear sharing agreement allows non-nuclear member countries to participate in planning and potentially deliver nuclear weapons in wartime. Approximately 100 US tactical nuclear bombs are deployed across five European NATO members: Belgium (20 at Kleine Brogel), Germany (20 at Büchel), Italy (40 at Aviano and Ghedi), the Netherlands (20 at Volkel), and Turkey (20 at Incirlik).

Even smaller countries possess these weapons of mass destruction. Belarus has begun hosting Russian tactical nuclear weapons. This widespread distribution of nuclear arsenals raises questions about the control and decision-making processes surrounding these weapons.

This list of nuclear weapon locations and incidents is far from complete. Many more accidents, both discovered and undisclosed, exist worldwide. The full extent of nuclear-related incidents in countries like Russia or China remains unknown. The sobering reality is that nuclear accidents can potentially occur anywhere, at any time, even in your backyard.

The nuclear arms race peaked in 1986. The Soviet Union had over 40,000 warheads, while the United States had 23,000. "Mutually assured destruction-fueled this buildup, as both sides believed arsenals would prevent attacks. Since the end of the Cold War, arms control agreements have been implemented.

The Nuclear Non-Proliferation Treaty began in 1970, the Strategic Arms Limitation Treaty in 1972, and the Strategic Arms Reduction Treaty in 1991. These treaties reduced nuclear arsenals. Some countries continue developing and modernizing their capabilities. France executed 210 tests, while the United Kingdom and China each conducted 45 tests. China's 1980 test was the last atmospheric detonation, and North Korea's 2017 underground test was the most recent. Some nations have dismantled their nuclear programs.

South Africa produced six nuclear weapons in the 1980s but dismantled them in the early 1990s. Belarus,

Kazakhstan, and Ukraine inherited Soviet weapons but transferred them to Russia by 1996. Nuclear weapon counts remain secret. The United States disclosed its stockpile size from 2010 to 2018.

This practice has become inconsistent recently. The United Kingdom stopped revealing figures for its arsenal in 2021, and other nuclear states provided minimal information. The global atomic weapon inventory is declining, and concerning trends have emerged. Reductions are slowing compared to previous decades. Military stockpiles are increasing again. China, India, North Korea, Pakistan, and Russia may be expanding their arsenals. Most nuclear-armed states are modernizing their weapons. This could increase the destructive power of existing arsenals.

Disarmament and non-proliferation efforts must continue. The international community needs to address nuclear weapon risks. A world without atomic annihilation threats remains a distant goal. Until then, we have enough nuclear weapons to blow up the entire planet many times over.

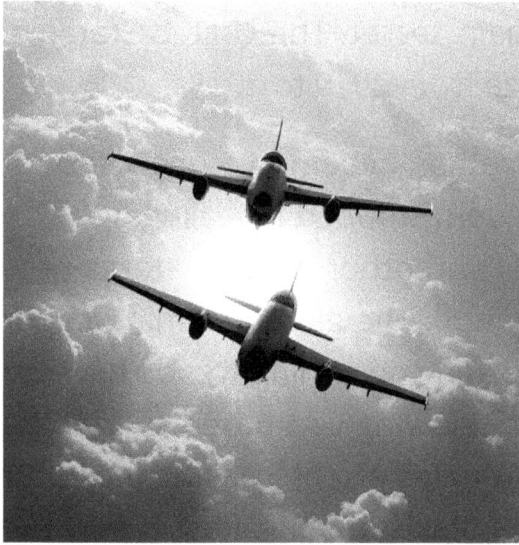

Chapter 7

The Razor's Edge

Throughout the Cold War and beyond, the world teeters on the brink of nuclear catastrophe far more often than most people realize. A series of close calls brings us close to global destruction. This chapter reveals lesser-known incidents that could have changed the course of history. It exposes the precarious nature of nuclear deterrence and the potential for errors to cause unintended catastrophes and even an extinction event.

On September 26, 1983, the Soviet nuclear early warning system Oko reported the launch of five intercontinental ballistic missiles from the United States. Lieutenant Colonel Stanislav Petrov, on duty at the Serpukhov-15 bunker near Moscow, suspected a false alarm. Petrov decided not to report the apparent attack to his superiors. His decision to wait for corroborating evidence prevented a retaliatory nuclear strike and averted a catastrophic nuclear war.

On November 9, 1979, computers at NORAD headquarters indicated that the Soviet Union launched 2,200 ballistic missiles toward the United States. This false alarm triggers a full-scale alert, with pilots scrambling to their jets. The panic lasted six minutes before officials determined it was a false alarm. The cause is a training tape simulating a Soviet attack mistakenly loaded into a critical computer system.

In November 1983, NATO conducted a military exercise called Able Archer 83, simulating a coordinated nuclear attack on Warsaw Pact countries. The realism of this exercise led Soviet leaders to believe it might be a ruse for an actual nuclear first strike. The Soviet military mobilized forces, transported nuclear weapons to launch sites, and prepared bombers carrying atomic warheads. The situation was defused when NATO concluded the exercise without incident, but the misinterpretation brought the world close to nuclear conflict.

On October 25, 1962, during the Cuban Missile Crisis, a guard at a U.S. military base in Duluth, Minnesota, spotted a figure scaling the fence. Alarms blared across the region, and at Volk Field in Wisconsin, a faulty system signaled nuclear-armed interceptors to scramble. The pilots rushed to their aircraft, believing nuclear war had begun. An officer raced onto the runway in his car, frantically flashing his lights to avert disaster.

During the Cuban Missile Crisis, Soviet submarine officer Vasili Arkhipov prevented a nuclear torpedo launch when U.S. destroyers cornered his submarine. His judgment under pressure saves millions of lives and prevents a rapid escalation of the conflict.

On May 23, 1967, a solar storm knocked out multiple NORAD radar systems across the Northern Hemisphere. Military officials initially interpreted this as Soviet jamming, an act of war. The nuclear missiles were almost launched.

In 1958, a B-47 bomber accidentally dropped a nuclear weapon into the waters off Tybee Island, Georgia. The bomb is never recovered, one of at least three "lost" U.S. nuclear weapons that remain unaccounted for today. These sunken relics of the Cold War can still be a potential for disaster lurking beneath the waves.

Although these events are not as severe as some historical incidents, they are worth noting. On January 25, 1995, Russian early warning systems detected a rocket launch off the coast of Norway. This was initially interpreted as a potential U.S. submarine-launched ballistic missile attack. The incident led to the activation of Russian nuclear forces, including the preparation of President Boris Yeltsinatomicear briefcase. The situation was de-escalated when it was confirmed that the rocket was on a Norwegian scientific mission to study the aurora borealis.

In June 2010, a U.S. missile defense test launch was misinterpreted by some observers as a potential ballistic missile threat. The test involved launching an interceptor missile from Vandenberg Air Force Base in California. While not a direct false alarm within military systems, the incident showed the potential for misinterpretation of missile launches, especially in regions with ongoing tensions.

On January 13, 2018, the Hawaii Emergency Management Agency mistakenly sent Hawaii residents a false ballistic missile alert. The alert, "BALLISTIC MISSILE THREAT INBOUND TO HAWAII. SEEK IMMEDIATE SHELTER. THIS IS NOT A DRILL," caused widespread panic. Although this was not an early military warning system error, it demonstrated the potential consequences of false alarms in the modern era of instant communication.

The USA almost attached itself. On January 23, 1961, a B-52 bomber carrying two Mark 39 hydrogen bombs broke apart over Goldsboro, North Carolina, with one bomb nearly detonating. On March 11, 1958, a B-47 bomber accidentally dropped a nuclear weapon over Mars Bluff, South Carolina, detonating conventional explosives and injuring people. These incidents highlight the dangers of transporting and handling nuclear weapons, even within a country's borders, and demonstrate the potential for harm even when weapons are not fully armed.

The United States and the Soviet Union actively suppress information about these near-catastrophic incidents. The Soviet Union denied the occurrence of the 1983 false alarm until 1998, long after the Cold War ended. The U.S. government keeps silent about these incidents, with much information remaining classified for decades. This mutual censorship underscores the high stakes and intense secrecy surrounding nuclear operations during the Cold War.

These incidents underscore the thin margin between peace and global destruction. They remind us of the danger posed by nuclear weapons and the importance of disarmament efforts. The fact that we avoid nuclear catastrophe owes much to luck and the systems in place. It remains a sobering thought in our still-nuclear world.

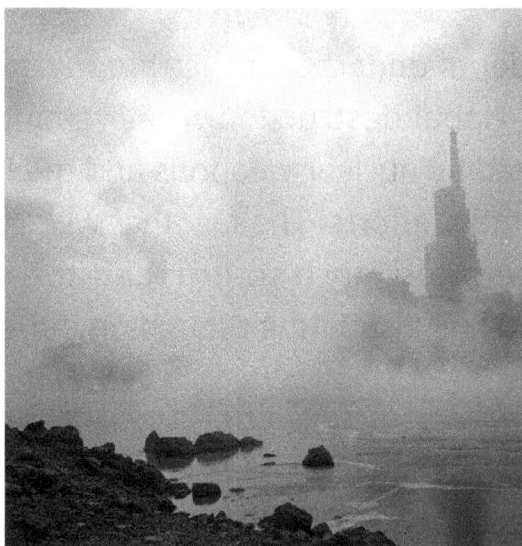

Chapter 8

Tritium The Added New Threat

T ritium is a radioactive isotope of hydrogen with one proton and two neutrons in its nucleus. It is produced artificially in larger quantities as a byproduct in all the world's nuclear reactors or through neutron bombardment of lithium; tritium is radioactive and emits weak beta radiation as it decays, with a half-life of 12.32 years.

Nuclear power plants release tritium into our environment through various pathways. Routine operations emit gaseous tritium into the air and discharge liquid effluents into water bodies. Leaks from corroded underground piping and equipment contaminate groundwater and soil, and spent fuel storage pools contaminate groundwater. The average nuclear power plant pressurized water reactor releases about 700 curies of tritium in liquid effluents annually.

The significance of these releases varies. At least 37 known and documented nuclear plant sites have experienced large tritium leaks exceeding federal drinking water standards, sometimes by hundreds of times. Many more undocumented cases likely exist among the 500 nuclear power plants and facilities worldwide. Most leaks remain contained on plant property. However, offsite contamination occurs, including contamination of private drinking wells near some plants. In the USA, about 30% of the population lives within 50 miles of nuclear reactors, which is easily within a Trituim exposure distance.,

The highest recorded tritium leak measured 15 million picocuries per liter—750 times the EPA drinking water limit. Exposure to such high levels could increase cancer risk. While the nuclear industry and regulators consider these releases of low safety significance, some experts and environmental groups argue that the standards are too permissive.

Tritium is released through cooling towers and cooling water systems. Airborne releases occur as water vapor from cooling towers disperses into the atmosphere. Waterborne releases occur when cooling water, used to condense steam from turbines, picks up tritium and returns it to the environment. In the United States, the Nuclear Regulatory Commission allows nuclear plants to release tritium, resulting in up to 100 milligrams per year of radiation dose to the public. The EPA's drinking water standard for tritium is 20,000 picocuries per liter.

European standards are more stringent, set by the European Union's drinking water directive. The E.U.'s directive sets a tritium limit of 100 Bq/L (about 2,700 picocuries per liter), lower than the US standard. This disparity raises questions about acceptable risk levels across nations and the role of regulatory bodies in setting these standards.

Ongoing monitoring and research continue to evaluate the potential long-term impacts of chronic low-level tritium exposure from nuclear plant releases. Tritium has a half-life of 12.32 years, decaying into helium-3. While it doesn't accumulate or become more potent over time, its effects on ecosystems are complex. Tritium enters the food chain through aquatic environments. Some become organically bound tritium (OBT) in tissues, with a longer biological half-life than tritiated water. Continuous release at the legal limit of 20,000 picocuries per liter maintains a relatively constant environmental level.

Authorities tell us that this legal limit of tritium is unlikely to directly kill fish or other aquatic organisms in the short term. However, the potential long-term impacts of chronic low-level tritium exposure are increased risk of genetic effects or cancer in organisms. So keep drinking that city water or healthy water near your nuclear power plants because you won't get sick immediately, just later.

Chronic exposure, even at permitted levels, may increase the risk of genetic effects or cancer in organisms over long periods. Different species exhibit varying sensitivities to tritium exposure. Regulatory limits include safety margins, but ongoing research evaluates the potential long-term impacts of chronic low-level exposure.

Tritium can accumulate in the environment and living organisms. It becomes part of the water cycle, persisting in ecosystems. Plants and animals incorporate it into organic molecules. Even at low levels, continuous exposure may increase long-term health risks. However, these risks are considered small at regulatory limits unless you live in the USA, where those limits are 641% higher than in Europe. (UE at 2700 vs. US at 20,000, which is 7,41 times higher or 641% higher)

The 'no threshold' model of radiation exposure suggests that any amount of radiation exposure carries risk. Tritium exposure poses health risks to everyone, particularly pregnant women and developing fetuses. This radioactive isotope emits beta radiation that can damage DNA, increasing cancer risk and causing genetic mutations. When ingested, tritium crosses the placenta, potentially affecting fetal development and leading to decreased body and brain weights in offspring. It can also impact fertility and damage organs like the liver and kidneys. While most tritium is eliminated from the body within weeks, some can become organically bound, contributing to long-term health risks. Regulatory limits aim to minimize these risks, but some experts advocate for stricter standards.

Laboratory detection limits range from 350 to 1000 picocuries per liter (pCi/L), above normal background levels. Due to the complexity of background levels and health risk thresholds, interpreting results often requires expert assistance. If tritium is detected, removing it from water is impossible using home treatment devices. The only effective method is to wait for radioactive decay.

Starting from the US limit of 20,000 pCi/L, levels would take 12 years to drop to 10,000 pCi/L, another 12 years to reach 5,000 pCi/L, and a further 12 years to get 2,500 pCi/L. This means 36 years is required for tritium levels to decay from the US discharge limit to near the European acceptable level. Are Americans more tolerant of nuclear contaminants in water? Who influences these regulatory decisions? Tritium has become a pervasive drinking water contaminant on Earth. This 'green' atomic energy is destroying our water supply and accumulating every day. We risk becoming the proverbial frog in slowly boiling water, unaware of the growing danger until it's too late.

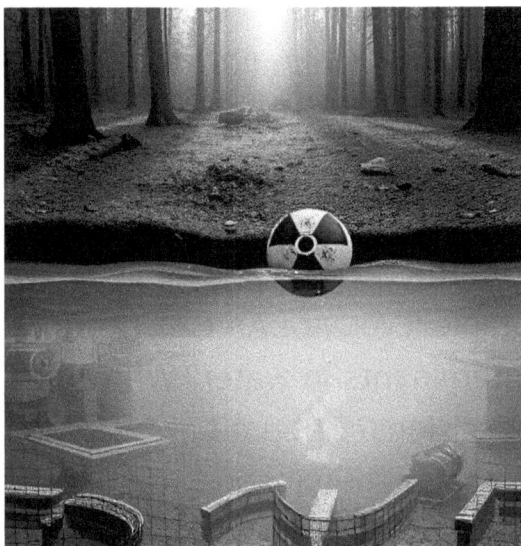

Chapter 9

Radioacitve Water Contaminaiton

Water contamination from radionuclides poses severe health risks. Radionuclides infiltrate water supplies and cause cancer, kidney damage, and developmental issues in animals and humans. Removing radioactive substances from water is nearly impossible, and prolonged exposure damages cells. People should avoid living near nuclear facilities and other locations that could release radionuclides.

The United States once had 100 nuclear power plants and other facilities. Many are now nearing the end of their intended design lives. Despite this, some plants have extended their design lives by 20 years. Numerous nuclear facilities have experienced radioactive releases, whether gas, liquid, or solid. Authorities often warn of potential releases only after they occur, leaving communities vulnerable.

In Miami, the Turkey Point facility has elevated salt, ammonia, phosphorus levels, and the radioactive tritium isotope in the water supply. These contaminants enter the aquifer, affecting millions of drinking water. The Vermont Yankee nuclear power plant has carcinogenic tritium in the groundwater. Oyster Creek in New Jersey and the Pilgrim Atomic Power plant in Massachusetts have also reported leaks. Once radionuclides enter water tables, they contaminate entire wells.

Radioactive isotopes, such as cesium-134, cesium-137, and iodine-131, can be absorbed through the skin, inhaled, or ingested and are linked to cancer. Atomic meltdowns, such as those at Three Mile Island and Fukushima, created plume clouds that dispersed radioactive isotopes. These isotopes entered the air, food, and water supplies, creating long-term health issues.

Cleaning isotopes from water is complex and nearly impossible. The half-life of uranium-235, found in nuclear weapons, is 703,800,000 years. Iodine-131, released from the Fukushima meltdown, has a half-life of eight days. Radium-226, found in Earth's crust, has a half-life of 1,600 years. Uranium-238, used in nuclear energy rods, has a half-life of 4,468,000,000 years. Protecting oneself from nuclear releases is difficult, especially if you live near any nuclear facility.

Fracking sites in America expose radioactive isotopes like radium-226, radium-228, uranium-238, and radon gas. These sites contaminate aquifers and water wells with chemicals, toxins, and radiation. Fracking creates chemical, biological, and radioactive waste, polluting potable resources. These wastes are toxic, radioactive, and often used as street deicing agents.

Nuclear facilities have had radioactive releases that contaminate water tables and supplies. The risk of radioactive contamination in aquatic life and fish is also a concern, as radiation leaks affect all marine life. When you eat fish, do you know where it came from? Is it radioactive?

Radiation dumping off the coast of New York City and California, along with the sinking of Russian nuclear submarines, adds to the contamination list. Due to these leaks, the fish we eat may be radioactive. As contamination increases, we may need to distill all our drinking water at home to ensure safety.

Distillation can effectively remove most radioactive contaminants from water, including uranium and radioactive fallout, by separating water from dissolved solids and killing biological pollutants. However, tritium, as discussed, is a radioactive isotope of hydrogen and cannot be removed because tritium behaves chemically like ordinary hydrogen in water molecules and will evaporate along with the water during distillation.

Personal Geiger counters may become necessary for monitoring radiation levels in everyday life. Buy one before the next disaster occurs today because they will be sold out.

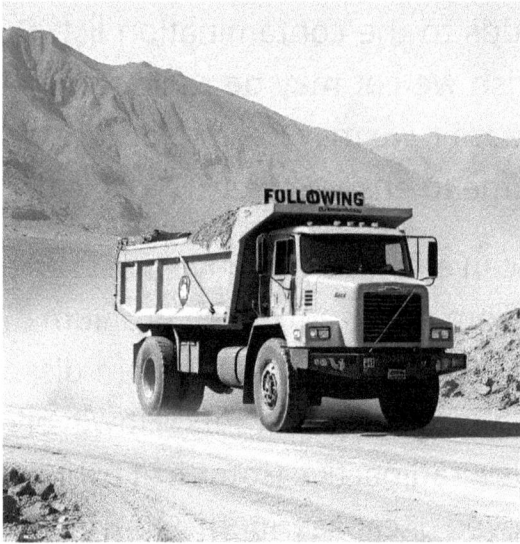

Chapter 10

One Of My Investigations

My investigation of a local radiation contamination site began when I learned about my father's early death at age 49. My father died of exposure to radioactive substances in the 1950s and during the Cold War. This revelation had a profound impact on me.

When I reached the same age, I started to awaken to the world's secrets and decided to conduct more research for my new project called "Erasing America." This project, intended as a YouTube channel, aims to uncover and document forgotten and abandoned sites with significant historical and environmental secrets.

For 15 years, I have traveled across the USA, exploring closed, abandoned, locked-down, and fenced-in sites. My investigations have covered various topics, including America's transformation due to big companies relocating to other countries. I visited abandoned sites like coal mines, shopping malls, garbage dumps, Geiger Counter manufacturers, hotels, high rises, superfund sites, and sites that contain hidden cold war nuclear secrets.

This story focuses on a site in my backyard, Cleveland, Ohio. When I first started visiting this site about twelve years ago, it was fenced off with barbed wire, non-operational, and guarded by security personnel. I would drive by day or night, noticing that the building next to Harvard Road always had lights on in one room on the second floor—a bizarre sight.

I contemplated sneaking into the site as I had done at other locations. However, my decision to refrain from trespassing proved wise when I uncovered the complex history of the property at the 1000 block of Harvard Avenue in Cleveland, Ohio. This location was once home to the Harshaw Chemical Company, a crucial contributor to the United States' nuclear program during the Cold

War era. The company's involvement can be traced back to World War II when the Manhattan Engineer District (MED) enlisted them to aid in the atom bomb project by developing uranium chemicals for the government.

From 1944 to 1959, Harshaw processed various forms of uranium at 1000 Harvard Avenue, Cleveland, Ohio. The uranium was then sent to Oak Ridge, Tennessee, for further processing. By 1949, Harshaw's Harvard Ave. facility had become one of the Manhattan Project's largest producers of uranium chemicals. The 55-acre Harshaw Chemical Company site, bordered by the Cuyahoga River and Big Creek, has been chemically manufactured since 1905. A 1984 radiological survey revealed extensive contamination throughout the site, with major contamination in Plant C and significant levels in 16 other buildings and 32 exterior locations. Soil samples indicated widespread contamination, including suspected contamination of the nearby river bed. The site contains long-lived isotopes like plutonium-239.

In December 2023, the U.S. Army Corps of Engineers awarded a $13.4 million contract for remedial action at Operable Units 1 and 2, including removing contaminated soil and debris related to FUSRAP. FUSRAP, or the Formerly Utilized Sites Remedial Action Program, is a federal initiative aimed at cleaning up sites contaminated with radioactive materials from the early atomic energy and weapons program.

Perhaps now is the opportune moment to begin my narrative about how this relates to the book. As a seasoned home inspector, I have thoroughly examined over 18,000 residences during my full-time career spanning four decades.

Thirty years ago, I checked a two-family house in a small neighborhood 1/4 mile from this Harshaw Plant area. During this inspection, one of the tenants in a two-family home I was inspecting told me they had cancer. Then, he said to me many other neighbors were sick and had cancers.

This information did not dawn on me, and I did not think much of it. Ten years later, I was doing another inspection in this area, and a home seller told me many people had cancers in this neighborhood.

When I read the newspaper article about constructing the metro park Bike Towpath, I read that this walking bike path had to stop because of an old Harshaw industrial site. The papers never came clean with all the details because Cleveland Newspapers always twisted or spun facts. This is a fact because they did it to me on numerous occasions. The Paper would take on my long, detailed new stories and cut out what they did not want, twist it, and skew it.

The contamination at the Harshaw Chemical Company site has impacted plans to extend the Ohio & Erie Canal Towpath Trail, part of the Cleveland Metroparks system. In January 2010, it was revealed the planned trail route crossed through radioactive land required cleanup to avoid long-term exposure hazards. This discovery forced planners to adjust the trail's path near the site.

Based on the information provided, the demolition of industrial buildings at the Former Harshaw Chemical Company site commenced in December 2014. From December 2014 to January 2015, the U.S. Army Corps of Engineers (USACE) dismantled contaminated and radioactive structures to facilitate further groundwater investigations beneath the building slab. The demolition began on December 26 amid freezing temperatures and a partially shut-down city due to Christmas Season.

Abatement contractors were tasked with spraying water to suppress dust during the demolition. Workers, clad in white hazmat suits and seemingly equipped with full-face respirators, operated machinery and performed their duties. When they noticed someone filming from the bridge, they halted operations and quickly moved towards several SUVs, presumably to investigate. However, the observer and that would be I swiftly departed the scene before they could be approached.

Approximately six months later, I observed soil loading from a stored pile left over from the winter's demolition. Intrigued, I followed the dump truck, leading me on an hour-long journey around the city. The driver seemed aware of my presence, deliberately taking a circuitous route.

Eventually, we returned to an area close to the original demolition site, about 10 minutes from where we had started at the Harshaw site. As we pulled into the E55th Street diner, I noticed the dump truck's load was uncovered. The driver exited the vehicle and fixed me with an intense stare, clearly aware that I had been tailing him.

Recognizing the potential danger, I quickly left the scene. The driver did not want me to discover the soil's final destination. After this unsettling encounter, I decided to cease my surveillance activities, realizing that pursuing this investigation further could put me at risk. Although I had a general idea of where the soil was being transported, I have remained silent about this incident ever since.

The entire nuclear industry is deceptive, sketchy, and secretive. Later, the EPA or environmental groups held a public meeting to discuss the future of this Harshaw Superfund site. Local news broadcasted this meeting only 15 minutes before it started at the Holiday Inn in a nearby suburb. I rushed to attend and found a room full of EPA officials, government representatives, and other nuclear officials. It felt as if all the attendees were actors, performing a routine they had done nationwide.

They staged the meeting as if many concerned citizens were present, but it seemed planned and orchestrated, complete with a PowerPoint presentation. I discreetly recorded parts of the meeting. Only three genuine attendees were present, including myself and two others, alongside about 20 individuals who appeared to be planted like seeds in a garden. A few contractors and EPA representatives were also in attendance, along with a projector for the presentation.

Government environmental groups discussed the site and their proposals, but to my knowledge, this information never made it to the headline news. The superfund cleanup team mentioned they would hold one more meeting, though I never received details about it. These types of meetings are common throughout the country and world, often appearing scripted and choreographed to give the illusion of public engagement.

The bottom line is that radiation was contained in the ground and groundwater, and authorities were concerned it might contaminate the City of Cleveland's stormwater supply. Since then, there has been radio silence. This is typical of the nuclear industry; they spin, choreograph, conceal, and effectively censor information from the public. Recently, I came across literature indicating that $13.5 million had been allocated to initiate a Superfund cleanup. Due to numerous projects and a busy life, I eventually stepped back from this surveillance project. However, curiosity recently led me to check on the site's progress. It appeared they were finally preparing for a Superfund cleanup.

On November 3, 2024, I visited the site and noticed a security guard in his car. While photographing EPA signs, the guard approached."What brings you here?" he inquired."Just taking pictures," I replied."For what purpose?""This is a contaminated Superfund site," I explained. The guard nodded. "I've heard about the contamination. That's why I'm here—I started this job three months ago, earning $26 an hour to watch the place. "Are you aware it's radioactive?" I asked."Some one mentioned it might be," he admitted.

Noticing his car parked on old foundations, I warned, "You should move your vehicle. It might not be safe there."Without hesitation, the guard rushed to relocate his car. Folks are still spinning, concealing, and lying... 80 years later. We will never know if the stormwater became contaminated or leaked into Lake Erie.

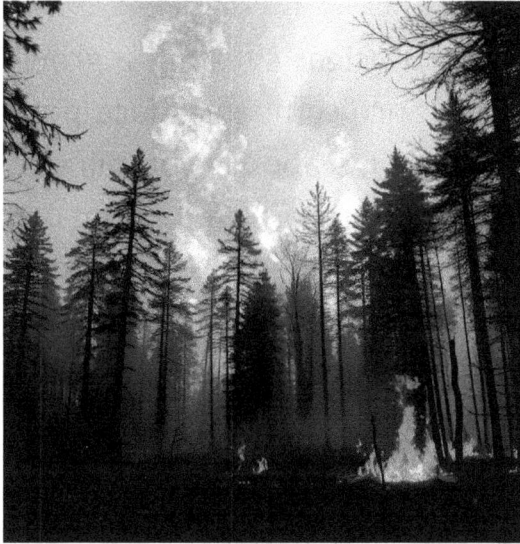

Chapter 11

Fires Unintended Consequence

N uclear accidents contaminate trees with radioactive isotopes, affecting wildlife and potentially spreading through forest fires. Smoke from these fires carries radioactive particles, impacting areas far from the source. Unreported fires in contaminated forests pose unknown risks to ecosystems and human health. This issue extends globally, with smoke from distant fires reducing visibility and air quality in cities thousands of miles away.

Forest fires near nuclear sites are a growing concern worldwide. Insurance companies face potential future challenges with claims about contamination from nuclear-affected forest fires. The full extent of this issue remains unclear due to limited reporting and documentation, which suggests the need for more comprehensive monitoring and research.

In the spring of 2023, smoke from Canadian fires reduced visibility in Cleveland, Ohio, to 1000 feet. These fires blanketed most of the upper part of North America with smoke. While gardening, I experienced contaminated breathing air firsthand. I went indoors and stayed indoors for the next five days. It was sad because millions contend with their daily routines, not even thinking of this potential threat. Authorities only reported particle size, not composition, leaving many questions unanswered.

Radioactive forest fires can spread contamination downstream, potentially contributing to long-term environmental impacts. The full effects of these Canadian fires on public health, both immediate and long-term, remain uncertain. Individuals with respiratory conditions or heart issues may have experienced increased symptoms in the weeks following the fires, but comprehensive data is lacking.

Now, let's discuss a small sample of 15 radioactive forest fires below, all lacking proper documentation. These cases illustrate the potential for unintended consequences from wildfires, especially those occurring in or near contaminated areas.

1969: Rocky Flats, Colorado, USA. The fire started on May 11, 1969, in Building 776-777 at Rocky Flats Plant due to spontaneous combustion of plutonium shavings in a glovebox. It burned through several hundred interconnected gloveboxes, causing extensive damage. The area contained plutonium-239 (half-life of 24,100 years) and plutonium-240 (half-life of 6,563 years) used in nuclear weapons production. Contamination spreads through improper storage and handling of radioactive materials. The fire released 13-62 millicuries of plutonium, contaminating areas southeast of the plant. It was the costliest industrial accident in U.S. history at the time, with damages estimated between $26-50 million.

2000: Cerro Grande Fire, New Mexico, USA. The fire started on May 4, 2000, in Bandelier National Monument as a prescribed burn that went out of control due to high winds and drought conditions. It burned 47,650 acres, including 7,500 acres within Los Alamos National

Laboratory. The area contained various radionuclides from decades of nuclear research and weapons development, including plutonium, uranium, and americium. Exact contamination levels were not publicly disclosed. The fire destroyed 235 homes in Los Alamos and damaged Laboratory structures. It increased runoff of radioactive contaminants, with plutonium transport downstream increasing 55 times compared to pre-fire levels.

2000: Hanford Site, Washington, USA. The 24 Command Wildland Fire started on June 27, 2000, from a fatal vehicle collision on State Route 24. It burned nearly 300 square miles, consuming an average of 2,000 acres per hour. The area contained various radioactive wastes from plutonium production for nuclear weapons. Major contaminants included plutonium-239 (half-life 24,100 years) and cesium-137 (half-life 30 years). The fire threatened several radioactive waste sites and the Fast Flux Test Facility. The fire passed over three inactive waste sites, and we do not have and reports of any radioactive releases.

2010: Mayak Nuclear Facility, Russia Wildfires broke out in the summer of 2010 near the Mayak facility in the Chelyabinsk region. The exact start date and cause are not specified in the provided sources. The area was contaminated from past nuclear accidents and routine releases from the Mayak facility. Major contaminants likely included strontium-90 (half-life 29 years) and cesium-137 (half-life 30 years). The fires raised concerns about the potential spread of radioactive contamination. Authorities hastily stripped vegetation from around the facility to prevent fire spread. Was that enough effort?

2011: Las Conchas Fire, New Mexico. The USA. The Las Conchas Fire started on June 26, 2011, in Santa Fe National Forest from a downed power line. It burned 156,593 acres, becoming the largest wildfire in New Mexico history. The area contained residual contamination from past nuclear research and testing at Los Alamos National Laboratory. Specific radionuclides and contamination levels were not detailed in the sources. The Las Conchas fire posed a significant threat to Los Alamos National Laboratory, advancing to within 3.5 miles of nuclear waste stored in temporary structures. This proximity increased the risk of radioactive contamination spread.

The Las Conchas fire intensified soil erosion and runoff, mobilizing contaminated materials. What is interesting is that the green environment is more worried about endangered species in New Mexico, including the Rio Grande Silvery Minnow, Southwestern Willow Flycatcher, Meadow Jumping Mouse, and Western Yellow-Billed Cuckoo than the humans that also live in this area.

2015: The Belarus-Ukraine border region. In 2015, fires occurred in radiation-contaminated forests along the Belarus-Ukraine border. The area was contaminated by the 1986 Chernobyl disaster, which contained cesium-137 (half-life 30 years) and strontium-90 (half-life 29 years). The fires caused resuspension and spread of radioactive particles.

2015: Chornobyl Exclusion Zone, Ukraine. Multiple fires broke out in the Chornobyl Exclusion Zone in 2015. The area was heavily contaminated by the 1986 reactor explosion, with cesium-137 and strontium-90 being significant contaminants. These fires burned through contaminated vegetation, releasing radioactive particles into the atmosphere. Mainstream news outlets never detailed the extent of radioactive spread and the environmental impact.

2017: Fukushima region, Japan. Wildfires occurred in areas contaminated by the 2011 Fukushima nuclear disaster in 2017. The region contained various radionuclides from the reactor meltdowns, including cesium-137 and iodine-131. These fires raised concerns about the potential spread of radioactive contamination through smoke and ash. The given sources did not provide specific details on the fires extent and radioactive releases.

2018: Chornobyl Exclusion Zone, Ukraine. Multiple fires again broke out in the Chornobyl Exclusion Zone in 2018. The area remained contaminated with long-lived radionuclides from the 1986 disaster. The fires burned through contaminated forests and vegetation, potentially mobilizing radioactive particles. The provided sources did not detail the extent of the fires and their impact on spreading radioactive contamination.

2018: Woolsey Fire, Southern California, USA. The Woolsey Fire started on November 8, 2018, burning 96,949 acres, including 80% of the Santa Susana Field Laboratory site. The lab was contaminated by a 1959 partial nuclear meltdown and rocket engine testing. The fire raised concerns about spreading radioactive contamination. Some studies found elevated levels of radioactive particles up to 9 miles from the site, while others reported no significant offsite contamination.

2019: Chornobyl Exclusion Zone, Ukraine. Fires occurred again in the Chornobyl Exclusion Zone in 2019. The area remained contaminated with long-lived radionuclides from the 1986 disaster, primarily cesium-137 and strontium-90. These fires burned through contaminated vegetation, potentially releasing radioactive particles into the atmosphere.

2020: Chornobyl Exclusion Zone, UkraineIn April 2020, major wildfires burned over 2,600 hectares of contaminated forest in the Chornobyl Exclusion Zone. The area contained various radionuclides from the 1986 disaster, including cesium-137 (half-life 30 years) and strontium-90 (half-life 29 years). Satellite imagery showed large plumes of smoke visible from space.

2022: Chornobyl Exclusion Zone, Ukraine. Seven wildfires broke out in the Chornobyl Exclusion Zone during the Russian invasion of Ukraine in 2022. The area remained contaminated from the 1986 disaster. These fires occurred during a period of military conflict, complicating firefighting efforts and raising concerns about potential radioactive contamination spread.

2024: Windy Deuce Fire, Texas, USA In 2024, the Windy Deuce Fire in Texas came within a few miles of the Pantex nuclear weapons facility. The facility contained various radioactive materials related to nuclear weapons production and maintenance. The fire necessitated the evacuation of non-essential employees from the Pantex facility.

These fires represent only a small sample of worldwide radioactive forest fires. We cannot control these fires or the events that cause them. These conditions can potentially materialize daily, as evidenced by recent wars or proxy wars.

Conflicts persist, with Ukraine facing radioactive contamination risks from fires in contaminated areas and forested regions. These fires act as derivatives of initial nuclear contamination, spreading radiation further. In this context, a derivative refers to an unintended consequence of an initial event.

Recent attacks have caused fires and destruction across Ukraine, potentially creating derivative radioactive dispersal. On November 3, 2024, a Russian drone attack ignited a fire in Kyiv's Shevchenkivskyi district. On November 11, Russian forces launched a massive assault on southern and eastern Ukrainian cities. These attacks caused fires and damage in Mykolaiv, Zaporizhzhia, and Kryvyi Rih, resulting in casualties and injuries.

Each fire in contaminated areas becomes a derivative event, spreading radioactive particles. Russia fired 145 drones at Ukraine over 48 hours, increasing derivative risks. Nuclear accidents contaminate land and forests worldwide. These contaminated areas face secondary disasters from accidents, weather events, and new wars, creating derivative scenarios.

The contamination spreads, initiating a chain of derivative events across the planet. Multiple nuclear accidents or releases occur globally, each with its consequences. These events intersect and amplify, contributing to potential extinction-level scenarios.

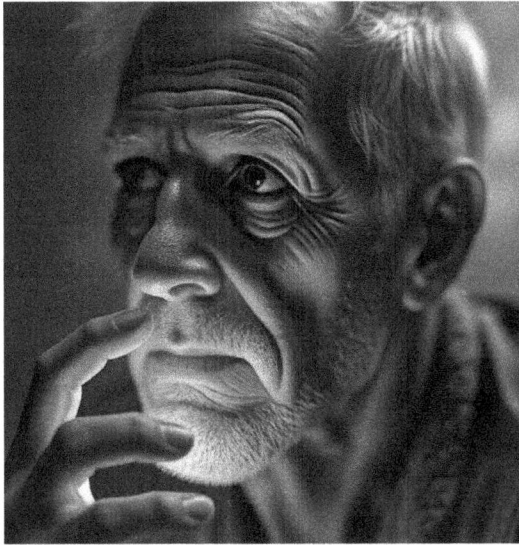

Chapter 12

Censorship, Compartmentalization, And Secrecy

The Manhattan Project, a secret U.S. World War II program, developed atomic bombs. It employed over 130,000 people across Los Alamos, Oak Ridge, and Hanford. Workers operated in compartmentalized secrecy, unaware of the project's full scope. The outcome was atomic bombs used on Hiroshima and Nagasaki in August 1945, causing Japan's surrender and ending World War II.

The bombings killed 140,000 in Hiroshima and 74,000 in Nagasaki by 1945's end. Survivors faced health effects, including cancer. Project workers exposed to radiation developed health issues. The project ushered in the nuclear age, impacting global politics and security. The Manhattan Project cast a dark shadow over nuclear history. Compartmentalization and secrecy shrouded the development of atomic weapons. Scientists and workers became unwitting sacrifices in the pursuit of nuclear power.

The Fukushima Daiichi disaster in 2011 had significant nuclear censorship. Japan's government monitored online reports and social media posts about the crisis, raising concerns about narrative control. Tokyo Electric Power Co. (TEPCO) admitted to delaying disclosure of meltdowns at three reactors for two months, describing it as "a cover-up." Japanese media reported heavy self-censorship on Fukushima-related topics due to pressure from the government and the nuclear lobby. In 2014, the newspaper Asahi Shimbun was forced to retract an article about the disaster, with journalists involved transferred or forced to resign.

The Kursk submarine disaster in 2000 saw the Russian government tightly control information, refusing to release a list of missing sailors, restricting media access, and heavily editing official broadcasts. In one instance, a distraught mother was forcibly sedated during a meeting with President Putin. These examples demonstrate various forms of information control, from direct government intervention to self-censorship and pressure on media organizations, in the aftermath of nuclear incidents.

The aftermath of the Fukushima disaster remains downplayed and censored. Specific individuals, like Dana Dunford and Kevin Blanch, face shadow banning or censorship for discussing anti-nuclear issues. Advocate voices are silenced to control the narrative. Even one of my anti-nuclear YouTube videos on my Clevelandmarko channel, which initially received over 60,000 views, dwindled to nothing. It's no accident.

Japan's request for elderly volunteers to clean up Fukushima went unreported. These volunteers died from radiation exposure, and their families were compensated in silence. Chernobyl's first responders met a similar fate, their sacrifices forgotten. Governments suppress damaging information about nuclear power. Authorities fear public awareness of its destructive potential and health risks. Radiation exposure limits in air, water, and soil are increased to accommodate industry needs.

The 2017 Mayak nuclear facility incident in Russia saw authorities initially denying the release of ruthenium-106 detected across Europe, later admitting to a release but downplaying its significance and refusing to disclose full details. In the same year, North Korea tightly controlled information about its nuclear test, releasing only carefully curated images and statements, forcing international observers to rely on seismic data and satellite imagery.

The International Atomic Energy Agency (IAEA) is the global nuclear watchdog established in 1957 to promote the safe and peaceful use of nuclear technology. It conducts inspections and verifications to ensure compliance with nuclear safeguards agreements.

The U.S. Department of Energy delayed reporting a tunnel collapse at the Hanford nuclear waste site, raising concerns about potential radiation releases. Iran has restricted IAEA inspections and controlled media coverage of its atomic activities, limiting transparency. Similar issues occurred during the Fukushima and Chornobyl incidents, where initial denials and restricted information hindered accurate risk assessment.

The biggest nuclear bomb detonated has the biggest concealment. The Soviet Union's detonation of the Tsar Bomba, the largest hydrogen bomb ever tested, on October 30, 1961, remained a closely guarded secret from its people for decades. This colossal 50-megaton device detonated over Novaya Zemlya in the Arctic Circle was approximately 3,333 times more prepotent than the Hiroshima bomb.

The Tsar Bomba created a fireball 5 miles in diameter with a mushroom cloud reaching 42 miles high. The explosion's effects were staggering, causing third-degree burns up to 62 miles from ground zero, destroying buildings 34 miles away, and shattering windows as far as Norway and Finland. The full details of this test and its consequences were only revealed to the Soviet public after the fall of the Soviet Union in 1991. This disclosure, along with information about other nuclear tests, sparked outrage among people in affected regions, particularly in Kazakhstan, where many Soviet atomic tests had been conducted.

While exact figures are difficult to determine due to the secrecy surrounding these tests, it is estimated that over the past 60 years, hundreds of thousands of people have been affected by the Soviet nuclear program. Studies suggest that approximately 1.5 million people in Kazakhstan alone were exposed to radioactive fallout, with many suffering from cancers, congenital disabilities, and other radiation-related illnesses. The full extent of the health and environmental consequences continues to unfold, affecting generations born long after the tests were conducted.

The nuclear industry's influence extends to media and policy. Opposition to nuclear power and uranium mining is systematically censored. This control of information aims to maintain public support for atomic energy. The actual cost of nuclear power remains hidden. Long-term environmental impacts are minimized or ignored. Health effects on communities near nuclear facilities are often dismissed or attributed to other causes.

Nuclear waste storage presents an unsolved problem. Governments struggle to find safe, long-term solutions. The risks of contamination persist for thousands of years, burdening future generations. Military applications of nuclear technology drive ongoing research and development. The threat of nuclear war looms while disarmament efforts stagnate. Proliferation concerns grow as more nations seek atomic capabilities.

The nuclear industry's economic viability relies on government subsidies and limited liability. Actual costs of accidents and waste management are externalized to taxpayers. This financial structure distorts the energy market. Uranium mining devastates landscapes and indigenous communities. Workers face occupational hazards, including increased cancer risks. These human and environmental costs are factored into nuclear energy discussions.

The nuclear weapons stockpile threatens global security. Modernization programs consume vast resources, perpetuating the arms race. Efforts to reduce atomic arsenals face political and technical issues. Radiation's invisible nature compounds public fear and mistrust. Governments and industry struggle to communicate risks. This information gap fuels conspiracy theories and undermines informed decision-making.

Nuclear technology's dual-use nature complicates international relations. Peaceful nuclear programs can mask weapons development. This ambiguity strains diplomatic efforts and non-proliferation agreements. The nuclear industry's influence extends to academia and research. Funding priorities control scientific inquiry and biasing results. Critical studies may face publication barriers or limited dissemination.

Nuclear accidents' long-term health effects remain understudied. Epidemiological research faces funding constraints and data access issues, hampering the proper assessment of atomic technology's true impact.

Decommissioning aging nuclear plants presents technical and financial burdens. The process takes decades and costs billions, soon trillions. Proper disposal of radioactive materials remains an unsolved problem. Nuclear energy's future remains uncertain. Public opinion shifts in response to accidents and environmental concerns, yet vested interests continue to promote nuclear power as a necessary energy source.

Nuclear censorship hides critical information about radiation releases, health risks, and environmental contamination from nuclear accidents and weapons production. This lack of transparency prevents people from taking protective actions, delays medical treatment for radiation exposure, and hinders efforts to clean up contaminated areas, ultimately endangering public health and damaging ecosystems.

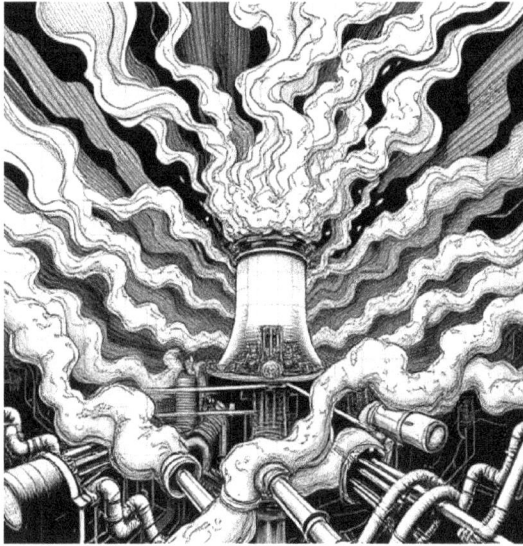

Chapter 13

The Radioactive Waste Is Pilling Up

N uclear waste storage problems plague the industry. Containers leak, solutions fail, and the waste keeps accumulating. Millions of fifty-five-gallon drums or one-ton storage bags, stored, buried, or submerged, rust, break, and release their deadly contents into the environment daily.

Superfund sites grow larger, defying cleanup efforts. Many radioactive substances have half-lives spanning millions of years. These sites remain hazardous for generations, with no viable long-term solution.

Hundreds of nuclear facilities worldwide store spent fuel rods on-site. They have nowhere else to send them. Some, like Fukushima, experienced catastrophic failures. Others use masonry block buildings, which are vulnerable to extreme weather events. A recent hurricane in the Carolinas may compromise several nuclear facilities. Mainstream media remains silent on these incidents. The public remains unaware of the potential dangers lurking in their communities.

Governments repurpose nuclear waste into armor-piercing munitions. These radioactive rounds litter battlefields across the globe. Congenital disabilities and deformities rise in affected areas yet receive little public attention.

Children in conflict zones unearth spent ammunition containing Uranium-235. This suggests the reprocessing of spent fuel rods into weapons. The practice spreads radioactive contamination far beyond nuclear facilities. Similar to this is the use of depleted uranium (DU) in munitions

Depleted uranium (DU) is a byproduct of uranium enrichment for nuclear fuel and weapons. Due to its high density and self-sharpening properties, it is widely used in armor-piercing ammunition. It is 40% less radioactive than natural uranium but still toxic as a heavy metal, and its density is 1.67 times greater than that of lead. DU is also pyrophoric, which ignites on impact, making it particularly effective in military applications.

The primary sources of DU are nuclear fuel production and spent fuel reprocessing, with the United States possessing large stockpiles from decades of nuclear programs. DU is commonly used in armor-piercing rounds for tanks, aircraft, and other vehicles, as well as tank armor for increased protection. Standard calibers for DU munitions include 20mm, 25mm, 30mm, and 120mm tank rounds.

Several countries, including the United States, United Kingdom, Russia, China, France, Pakistan, and Israel, have incorporated DU munitions into their military arsenals. These weapons have been used in various conflicts, such as the Gulf War (1991), Bosnia (1994-1995), Kosovo (1999), and the Iraq War (2003). NATO countries with compatible weapons systems have also received DU ammunition, and recently, the use of DU rounds was approved for Ukraine with U.S.-supplied Abrams tanks.

Despite its military effectiveness, the use of DU munitions remains controversial due to potential health and
environmental risks. Concerns include soil and water
contamination, kidney damage, and increased cancer
risk from inhaling DU dust. The long-term impacts of
DU use are still debated within the scientific community.
While exact numbers of DU rounds produced and used
are classified, estimates suggest that millions have been
manufactured and possibly a million have been used in
conflicts.

Many countries are now littered with radioactive buried
bullets that have a half-life of millions of years. Children
find these and play with them. We give these to other
countries like Ukraine today so they can continue their
war and contaminate the land of Russia, where children
may unearth and play with them in the future. This situation is insane and makes no sense. Our world is turning
into that future dystopia called "Idiocracy," where they
feed vegetation and farm animals Gatorade.

The threat of nuclear terrorism looms. In 1961, a U.S.
B-52 carrying atomic weapons crashed near Goldsboro,
North Carolina. One bomb almost detonated on the
land that built it. How insane can this nuclear dilemma
get? Are all these theories fundamental? Remember
the whole thing about "Weapons of Mass Destruction"
that led the USA on a wild goose chase, killing leaders

and bombing the world? Is this reality or an illusion or deception to control the masses? We watch this stuff or let's call it propaganda, all day, and we believe it.

Nuclear power energy has many harmful aspects. These include bombs, mining, storage, deployment, leaks, energy, submarines, ships, and waste management. It destroys wildlife, plants, and humans. Contaminated areas remain uninhabitable for centuries. The actual cost of atomic power is immense. It goes far beyond electricity generation.

Our leaders and conglomerates seem psychopathic and insane. They're trying to decommission old, radioactive power plants while building new "future dinosaurs." These are supposedly more efficient nuclear power plants. They're being constructed worldwide, even on movable ships. If one leaks on a ship, we might never know.

Today, we already have 437 operational nuclear power reactors worldwide, with an additional 59 under construction. Even more concerning, plans for approximately 96 more reactors are in various planning stages. It's as if we're touching a hot stove repeatedly despite knowing the consequences.

The nuclear industry's push for expansion seems to ignore the lessons learned from past disasters like Chornobyl and Fukushima. These new plants are touted as safer and more efficient, but they still pose significant risks and generate radioactive waste that will remain dangerous for thousands of years.

The nuclear industry struggles to contain its toxic legacy. Waste piles up with no permanent storage solution. Future generations will bear the burden of our atomic decisions. Depleted uranium munitions pose health risks to soldiers and civilians alike: heavy metal toxicity and radiation exposure cause organ damage, neurological problems, and congenital disabilities.

Veterans returning from wars often face high rates of illness and suicide due to mental health issues like PTSD, traumatic brain injuries, difficulty accessing care, and problems readjusting to civilian life. Radiation exposure can be one of the reasons for some veterans' health issues, especially those exposed during nuclear testing or cleanup operations and handling radioactive munitions such as armor-piercing bombs and bullets.

Studies show increased cancer rates and congenital disabilities in areas where depleted uranium weapons were used. The debate over long-term health effects continues, with conflicting scientific reports. The nuclear industry relies on government subsidies and limited liability. Taxpayers bear the actual costs of accidents and waste management. This financial structure distorts the energy market.

Decommissioning aging nuclear plants presents technical and financial hurdles. The process takes decades and costs hundreds of billions and possibly trillions. Proper disposal of radioactive materials remains an unsolved problem. Nuclear energy's future remains uncertain—public opinion shifts in response to accidents and environmental concerns, yet vested interests continue to promote nuclear power as a necessary energy source.

The nuclear waste dilemma persists. No country has successfully implemented a permanent solution, and temporary storage facilities are filling up, creating new risks and issues. Radiation's invisible nature compounds public fear and mistrust. Governments and industry struggle to communicate risks effectively. This information gap fuels conspiracy theories and undermines informed decision-making.

Nuclear technology's dual-use nature complicates international relations. Peaceful nuclear programs can mask weapons development. This ambiguity strains diplomatic efforts and non-proliferation agreements. The nuclear industry's influence extends to academia and research. Funding priorities change scientific inquiry, potentially biasing results. Critical studies may face publication barriers or limited dissemination.

As nuclear waste accumulates, the search for safe, long-term storage continues. The clock ticks on this radioactive time bomb, threatening future generations with a toxic inheritance.

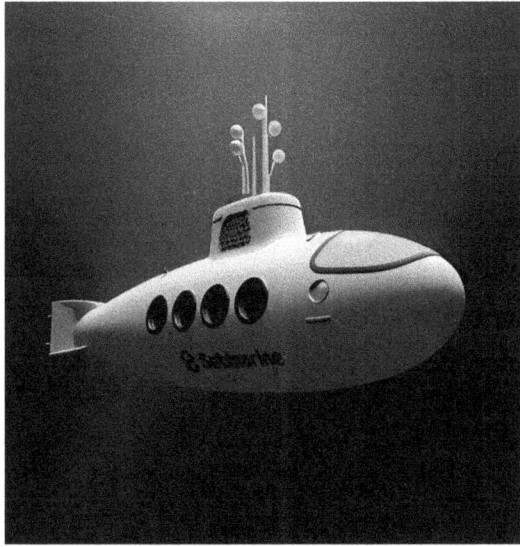

Chapter 14

Nuclears Submerines And Ships.

N uclear submarines emerged as naval warfare machines in the 1950s with the launch of the USS Nautilus, which introduced enriched uranium reactor technology. The U.S. took the lead, building 245 nuclear submarines by the 1990s. Russia joined the race in 1958 with the K-3 Leninskiy Komsomol. Today, the U.S. has 66+ active-duty atomic submarines, and Russia has 30.

The UK, France, China, and India also developed atomic submarine capabilities. The proliferation of nuclear submarines led to establishing international treaties and agreements to regulate their use and disposal. However, with nuclear reactors in submarines having a very short lifespan of 10 to 33 years and no clear end-game plans, the inevitable threat is undeniable.

Since 1950, hundreds of these nuclear dinosaurs have been manufactured and thrown into our oceans. According to some international agreements, Russia decommissioned 200 atomic submarines, the U.S. 100, and France 25. Decommissioning involves removing the nuclear fuel and other hazardous materials and dismantling the reactor and other components. Russia dismantled 100, France dismantled 11. The U.S. lost two submarines at sea, France lost 7. The Washington Hanford nuclear graveyard houses ten additional old submarines for future decommissioning.

The Cold War mishaps sunken submarines all over the world are now rusting, leaking, and killing our oceans. The USS Thresher sub sank in 1963, claiming 129 lives. The USS Scorpion followed in 1968, with 99 lost. Russia's losses include K-8 in 1970 and K-278 Komsomolets in 1989. The Kursk tragedy in 2000 took 118 lives. These underwater tombs are active environmental hazards, leaking radioactive materials into the ocean

NUCLEAR EXTINCTION EVENT IS KILLING OUR FAMILIES

and contributing to the deterioration of marine ecosystems, along with rotting human bodies.

Decommissioned vessels face different fates on land—the Hanford Site in Washington stores 144 submarine reactor compartments along collapsing tunnels full of train cars full of radioactive waste. This Hanford place is so radioactive that sometimes you cannot even fly overhead planes. Russia's Kara Sea graveyard holds 14 reactors and a crippled submarine. These sites are huge, substantial graveyards. This term describes sites contaminated with hazardous substances that create havoc on human health, plant life, and our entire planet.

Sunken submarines eventually leak radiation into oceans. In some areas, the K-278 Komsomolets show radiation levels 800,000 times higher than usual. Recently, K-159, which sank in 2003, will continue to leak and be radioactive for millenniums.

Russia identified only six sunk submarines, and many more exist in the Arctic oceans. These vessels contain Radioactive isotopes like cesium-137 and strontium-90 and have 30-year half-lives. Today, models predict increased cesium levels in cod and other marine foods we consume. When our media shows us skinny, starving polar bears, are they emaciated polar bears with leukemia?

During the Cold War, many submarines carried nuclear propulsion systems and weapons. Several of these submarines sank. The Soviet submarine K-278 Komsomolets sank in 1989. It had two nuclear warhead-armed torpedoes. The USS Scorpion, an American submarine, was lost in 1968. It carried nuclear-tipped Mark 45 torpedoes. These sunken submarines pose environmental risks. They could leak radioactive materials into the ocean. The Soviet K-219 and K-129 submarines also carried nuclear armaments when lost at sea.

These sunken submarines continue to pose potential environmental hazards due to the risk of radioactive leakage from both their nuclear reactors and weapons. The Komsomolets wreck, for instance, is still monitored for possible contamination. The presence of nuclear materials in these sunken vessels has complicated salvage efforts and raised long-term concerns about the impact on marine ecosystems.

Nuclear submarines utilize pressurized water reactors (PWRs) for propulsion, employing enriched uranium as fuel. These reactors heat water in a closed primary loop, transferring energy to a secondary loop to generate steam for turbines. The main fissile isotope, uranium-235, has a half-life of about 704 million years, ensuring long-term power generation for the submarine. However, this also means the radioactive waste produced will remain hazardous for a long time.

When a nuclear submarine sinks and when the reactor containment breaks, radioactive material leaks into the ocean. This will happen 100% before the 704 million half-life, causing genetic mutations and health issues to affect populations worldwide.

Nuclear-powered surface ships have been a significant part of naval fleets since the Cold War era. The United States currently operates 11 nuclear-powered aircraft carriers, while Russia maintains a fleet of nuclear-powered icebreakers and has recently deployed a floating nuclear power plant. At the end of the Cold War, the US also had nine nuclear-powered cruisers, which have since been decommissioned. Russia has decommissioned some of its older nuclear icebreakers, including at least two from the Arktika class.

These nuclear-powered vessels pose potential environmental and health risks, particularly when they are decommissioned or if they sink. The consequences could be severe in the event of war or other disasters that could cause these ships to sink,

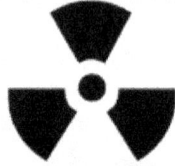

DANGER

RADON GAS

Chapter 15

Radon

The Silent Threat Radon is a radioactive gas formed from the decay of uranium in soil and rock. It seeps into buildings through cracks and openings and becomes trapped inside. This colorless, odorless gas is the second leading cause of lung cancer in the United States after smoking.

The Environmental Protection Agency estimates radon causes 21,000 lung cancer deaths annually. Smokers exposed to radon face a much higher risk of developing lung cancer than non-smokers. Radon can accumulate in any building, including homes, schools, and offices.

Modern construction techniques have increased indoor radon levels. Energy-efficient homes with tight seals and improved insulation trap more radon inside. Negative air pressure from HVAC systems can draw additional radon from the ground into living spaces.

Building materials like concrete, granite, and wallboard can emit radon. Granite countertops, popular in kitchens and bathrooms, may release small amounts of radon gas. These materials can also cause elevated radon levels in high-rise office buildings. Since the COVID-19 pandemic, Americans have spent over 80% of their time in their homes. This increased indoor time, combined with tighter building envelopes, means people breathe more radioactive air now then in the past.

Water supplies can contribute to indoor radon levels. Groundwater from deep wells often contains dissolved radon, which is released into the air during household use. Showering, washing dishes, and doing laundry can all release radon from water into the home.

Certain occupations carry a higher risk of radon exposure. Uranium miners, phosphate fertilizer handlers, and workers in underground spaces face increased radon levels. Consumer products like radioluminescent watch dials and firearm sights can contain small amounts of radon precursors.

Outdoor air has lower radon concentrations than indoor air. However, local geology and weather patterns can affect outdoor radon levels. Some areas have higher radon concentrations due to underlying rock formations rich in uranium. Fracking byproducts used as de-icing agents on roads can contain radon. As these materials break down, they may release radon into the environment. This practice adds another potential source of radon exposure to daily life.

Radon awareness and testing have increased in recent years. The EPA's 1992 estimate of 1 in 15 homes having high radon levels is likely underestimated today. Improved detection methods and more frequent testing reveal the widespread nature of this issue.

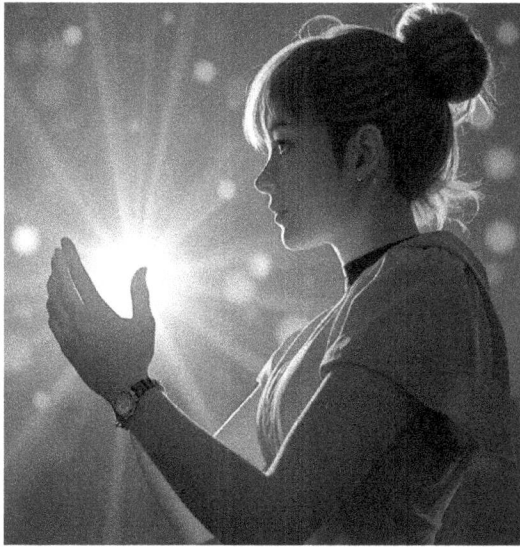

Chapter 16

Fighing Cancer With Cancer

C ancer rates have risen dramatically over the past century. In 1900, approximately 3% of the population was diagnosed with cancer. By 1960, this figure had increased to 7%. In 2024, cancer affects nearly 40% of people during their lifetime. Ironically, radiation therapy remains a standard cancer treatment. This approach essentially fights cancer with another carcinogen. The medical community justifies this method as necessary to combat advanced tumors.

The overall health of populations continues to decline. Chronic illnesses, autoimmune disorders, and unexplained ailments are becoming more prevalent. These conditions may be precursors to cancer or independent effects of radiation exposure.

Radiation exposure causes more than just cancer. It can lead to genetic mutations, organ damage, and cognitive impairment. Many of these effects go undiagnosed or are attributed to other causes. The impact of radiation can take decades to manifest. Survivors of nuclear incidents often develop health problems years or even generations later. This delayed onset complicates efforts to link illnesses directly to radiation exposure.

Radiation therapy can cause secondary cancers by damaging DNA in healthy cells, leading to genetic mutations that may result in malignant transformation years after treatment. Additionally, radiation exposure can cause other health problems like tissue damage, organ dysfunction, and increased risk of cardiovascular disease, with the severity and likelihood of these issues depending on factors such as radiation dose, treatment area, and individual patient characteristics.

Hospitals and dental offices routinely use radiation in diagnostic and therapeutic procedures, exposing patients to varying radiation levels. The health effects of radiation depend on the dose received, with exposure to 100 mSv increasing cancer risk by 0.5%, while 1,000 mSv causes radiation sickness. More severe effects occur at higher doses: 5,000 mSv is lethal for 50% of people within a month, and acute exposure to 10,000 mSv causes death within weeks. For context, natural background radiation averages 2-3 mSv per year.

Radiologic technologists face cumulative radiation exposure over their careers. Studies show that technologists receive higher doses than the public. The median annual dose for fluoroscopically guided procedures is 0.65 mSv. Long-term effects include increased cancer risk for technologists working before modern safety standards.

Hospital treatments are at lower levels with associated exposures: chest X-ray: 0.1 mS; Mammogram: 0.4 mSv; Head CT scan: 2 mSv; Abdominal CT scan: 10 mSv; Coronary CT angiogram: 16 mSv; PET/CT scan: 25 mSv; and Radiation therapy for cancer: 20-80 Gy (20,000-80,000 mSv) to the tumor site. Radiation is never a sure bet; even at low dosages, injury can result.

CT scans and high-radiation imaging procedures raise concerns about unnecessary patient exposure. These scans provide valuable diagnostic information but have higher radiation doses than conventional X-rays. A single CT scan exposes a patient to 1-10 mSv, equivalent to hundreds of chest X-rays.

Dental X-rays raise concerns due to potential overexposure and health impacts. Studies link frequent dental X-rays to increased cancer risks, particularly in children and adolescents. Dental radiography in the U.S. may contribute to nearly 1,000 excess cancer cases annually.

Radiation treatment does not always add years to life for cancer patients. The impact on life expectancy varies depending on cancer type, stage, and other treatments. For non-small cell lung cancer, radiation therapy improves overall survival across all stages. Nobody accumulates or counts an entire life of radiation treated or exposed. Radiation-related illnesses remain underreported due to limited awareness.

A 72-year-old patient's lifetime radiation exposure from medical imaging includes 200 dental X-rays (1 mSv), 10 CT scans (100 mSv), and 20 chest X-rays (2 mSv), totaling 103 mSv. This exceeds the recommended occupational exposure limit of 100 mSv over 5 years. Additional exposure sources include radioactive granite countertops, consuming radioactive salmon, overhead power lines, and other environmental factors. These cumulative exposures are not typically tracked or measured, potentially leading to underestimated total radiation exposure over a lifetime.

These medical uses of radiation are carefully controlled and prescribed only when the diagnostic or therapeutic benefits may outweigh the small risks associated with exposure. Healthcare providers adhere to the ALARA principle (As Low As Reasonably Achievable) to minimize unnecessary radiation exposure while achieving the necessary clinical outcomes. This approach ensures patients receive the benefits of these essential medical procedures while keeping radiation risks as low as possible. However, other radiation treatments exist that are not controlled.

Radioactive hot springs were popular health destinations. Visitors bathed in and drank radioactive water, believing it had healing properties. Some spas, like Joachimsthal, exposed patrons to doses of up to 7 mSv per hour. Even today, radiation therapy is used in several unconventional treatments, including radon spas in Austria and Germany, where patients bathe in radon-rich water to alleviate pain from conditions like arthritis. In Ukraine, people take radon baths to treat various ailments, including back injuries and infertility.

Some clinics offer thorium-containing "monazite sand baths" for supposed health benefits. Low-dose radiation therapy is sometimes used to treat non-malignant conditions like plantar fasciitis.

Some people visit Japan's radioactive hot springs called "onsen" for their healing properties. However, these practices come with significant risks. Exposure to radon and other radioactive substances increases cancer risk, particularly lung cancer. The perceived benefits are often not scientifically proven, and pain relief may be temporary or due to placebo effects. Long-term exposure to even low doses of radiation can lead to DNA damage and increased cancer risk. Additionally, these treatments may delay people from seeking evidence-based medical care for their conditions.

Radiation alters DNA in all living organisms. Plants, insects, and animals near contaminated sites exhibit genetic abnormalities. These changes can persist and spread through ecosystems long after the initial exposure.

The disposal of radioactive medical equipment poses significant risks. In one incident, contaminated metal from Mexican hospitals was recycled into building materials, and these radioactive studs ended up in homes across the United States. Radioactive medical equipment being recycled and unknowingly put back into public use has led to several dangerous incidents. In Samut Prakan, Thailand (2000), an unlicensed cobalt-60 radiation source from medical equipment was recovered by scrap metal collectors, resulting in 10 hospitalizations and three deaths. A similar incident occurred in Goiânia, Brazil (1987) when scavengers broke open an abandoned radiation therapy machine containing cesium-137, leading to 250 people being contaminated and four deaths. In Mexico (2013), a truck transporting a cobalt-60 teletherapy source from a hospital was stolen, risking public exposure before authorities recovered it.

Other incidents include the 2010 Mayapuri, India case, where a research irradiator containing cobalt-60 from Delhi University was auctioned to a scrap market, resulting in 7 people being exposed to radiation and one death. This is just one of many events that result from the improper disposal or theft of radioactive medical equipment, leading to unintended public exposure and potentially severe health consequences.

In 1983, a radiation therapy machine was scrapped in Ciudad Juarez, Mexico, and its cobalt-60 source melted into steel. Contaminated rebar was used in building construction. Some homes still contain radioactive materials, exposing residents to elevated radiation levels. From 1982 to 1984, recycled steel contaminated with cobalt-60 was used to construct over 1,700 apartments in Taiwan. Residents were exposed to radiation levels of up to 600 mSv per year, increasing cancer risks.

In 2000, in the Lia radiological incident in Georgia, three lumberjacks found abandoned Soviet radioisotope thermoelectric generators in the forest. They suffered acute radiation sickness from cesium-137 exposure, receiving doses between 2,000 and 4,000 mSv.

Let's look at a few other types of radiation exposure anomalies—just a short list on the Internet. I can assure you that thousands of these stories exist, and most are not documented or unknown.

In the early 1900s, radium was hailed as a miracle cure. Companies sold radium-infused products like toothpaste, suppositories, and drinks. Eben Byers consumed 1000 bottles of radium water for health benefits. He died from radiation poisoning and was buried in a lead-lined coffin. What about the other thousand that drank this radioactive position

Shoe-fitting fluoroscopes were common in shoe stores from the 1920s to the 1950s. Customers placed their feet inside the machine, exposing them to harmful X-rays. In one case, a child received a dose of 116 mSv during a single fitting, leading to significant illness a year later. What about the thousands of other customers who were exposed? The next time your dentist wants to take the four yearly teeth X-rays, consider saying, "No, not this year." I don't let my dentist do this anymore unless it is essential. Sadly, dental insurance often won't pay unless you have X-rays.

After a B-52 bomber collision in Spain in 1966, locals collected radioactive debris as souvenirs. Many suffered radiation sickness from exposure to plutonium, with some receiving doses exceeding 250 mSv. In 1987, in Goiânia, Brazil, scrap metal scavengers found a discarded radiotherapy unit containing caesium-137. They took it home and distributed the glowing blue powder. Two hundred fifty people were contaminated, with four fatalities. Some individuals received doses of up to 7,000 mSv. In Taiwan, between 1982 and 1984, recycled steel contaminated with cobalt-60 was used to construct over 1,700 apartments. Residents were exposed to radiation levels of up to 600 mSv per year.

Radioactive isotopes were also put in children's toys, as exemplified by the Gilbert U-238 Atomic Energy Lab. Released in 1950 by the A.C. Gilbert Company, this controversial educational toy contained radioactive materials, including four uranium ore samples, a Geiger counter, a cloud chamber, and other nuclear physics equipment. Marketed as a safe and educational tool to teach children about atomic energy, the kit sold for $49.50 (equivalent to about $630 in 2023) and was accompanied by a comic book titled "Learn How Dagwood Splits the Atom."

Despite the company's claims of safety, backed by Oak Ridge Laboratories, the toy has since been criticized for its potential dangers. Radar Magazine dubbed it one of "the ten most dangerous toys of all time" in 2006. The kit was commercially unsuccessful, with fewer than 5,000 units sold during its brief production run in 1950 and 1951. While there are no widely reported cases of illness directly attributed to the toy, health and safety concerns ultimately led to its removal from the market in 1952. Today, these rare kits are sought-after collector's items, fetching prices as high as $5,000.

Other toys and children's products were radioactive, reflecting a time when the dangers of radiation were not fully understood or downplayed. Radium-based glow-in-the-dark products were trendy, and many toys and watches featured radium paint to create a luminous effect. These included clock faces, instrument dials, and children's toys like marbles, balls, and playing cards.

When my brother and I were 7 and 6, we found a glow-in-the-dark ball and cut it open. Fascinated by the glowing liquid inside, we painted our faces with it, un-aware of its dangers. We scared our grandmother, who freaked out and threw us into the shower. Thank you, Starimama (RIP). Ironically, this happened while our father was dying in Arizona from leukemia caused by his work at GE Nela Park, where he helped invent radioactive light bulbs.

The ball contained a mixture of radium salts and zinc sulfide, a common practice for creating self-luminous toys in the early 20th century. This radioactive compound emitted a continuous glow without needing to be charged by light. My brother died at 60, and while I'm still alive, I'll never know the full impact of our childhood exposure to this hazardous substance. According to resources, we were exposed to 25 mSVe to 300 mSv, 100x the acceptable yearly human dosage.

The Atomic "Bomb" Ring, introduced in 1947 as a Kix cereal premium, contained a tiny amount of polonium-210 and allowed children to see scintillations caused by radioactive decay. Soon after killing hundreds of thousands of Japanese people with an Atomic Bomb, this company manufactured these children's ring toys.

Even household items weren't exempt from this trend. Fiestaware, a famous brand of ceramic dinnerware, used uranium oxide in its glazes to produce vibrant orange-red colors from the 1930s to the 1970s. While not a toy, the Navigator, a 1920s-era water crock lined with radium, was marketed as a health product for families, claiming to add beneficial radioactivity to drinking water. These products demonstrate how radioactive materials were casually incorporated into everyday items, including those meant for children's use.

I bought some of this glass and used a Geiger counter to make several YouTube videos about ten years ago, which can still be found on my YouTube channel, CleavelandMarko. These experiments allowed me to demonstrate firsthand the radioactive properties of uranium glass. Using a UV light, I showcased the glass's distinctive green glow, a telltale sign of its uranium content. The Geiger counter readings provided tangible evidence of the low-level radiation emitted by this green glass.

If you're my age or older, you probably had one of those glow-in-the-dark alarm clocks. These tiny white clocks hummed and emitted a significant electromagnetic field. What about the millions of people who owned these? The Western Clock Manufacturing Company, known as Westclox, was a significant producer of these clocks. Founded in 1888, Westclox became famous for its Big Ben and Baby Ben models, selling over 50 million units by the early 1960s.

Their clocks were famous for their functionality and luminous dials that glowed in the dark, making them a staple in many households. However, the electromagnetic fields (EMF) these clocks emit have raised concerns about potential health risks. Studies have shown that prolonged exposure to EMF may be linked to various health issues, including sleep disturbances and increased cancer risk. While many people enjoyed the convenience of these clocks, the long-term effects of EMF exposure remain a topic of discussion. Reflecting on my childhood experiences with that clock and painting my faces with radioactive isotopes, I wonder how it may have impacted my health.

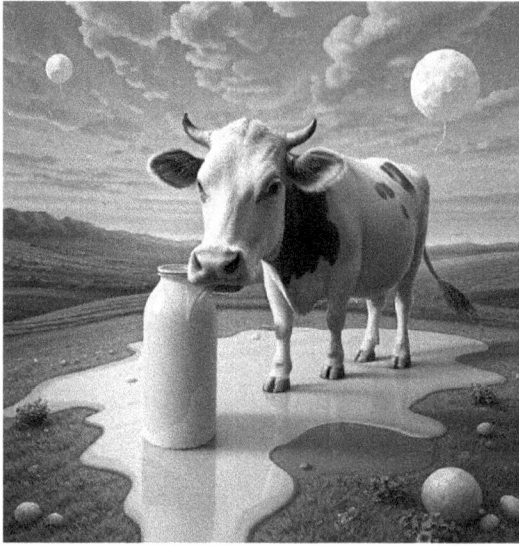

Chapter 17

Radioative Milk Testing

The Fukushima Disaster occurredo on March 11, 2011. The meltdown explosion produced a radioactive plume cloud that traveled across the Pacific Ocean and covered the world for many weeks. Authorities tested milk in Hawaii on March 4, 2022. Cows react first to radioactive fallout. Tests found radioactive strontium, cesium, and iodine isotopes. Officials claimed these were low-level. After Hawaii's milk tests, many USA cities stopped testing milk.

Today, Hawaii has higher overall cancer incidence rates than the U.S. average, ranking 5th highest for breast cancer incidence. The state's cancer burden varies by specific cancer type, with higher rates for liver, stomach, breast, and uterine cancers but lower rates for lung, bladder, brain, and leukemia compared to national averages.

No safe level of radionuclide exposure exists, whether from food, water, or other sources. Exposure to iodine-131, cesium-137, cesium-134, and strontium isotopes increases cancer risk. USDA cows pastured, ate, and drank in American fields during this period. The EPA shut down some radiation testing. Authorities should have reported on monitoring radiation detections.

In 2011, the EPA conducted radiation fallout tests at more than 100 locations in the USA, equating to one test every 24,000 square miles. However, the EPA failed to report detections, leaving the public uninformed about the extent of the contamination. The EPA also failed to inform or detect radioactive isotopes, including iodine, cesium, and strontium, that settled from clouds covering much of America's surface.

These beta isotope daughters had half-lives of 60 days or less, while uranium and plutonium have half-lives of thousands of years. In meltdowns, uranium and plutonium stay local. The Fukushima explosion created beta radiation isotopes, which travel high into the sky's jet stream. The radiation of these beta isotopes diminishes by 50% every sixty days, peaking from March through September 2011.

Fukushima's radioactive meltdown exposed American beef to fallout. Five days later, wind and jet stream dumped it on the USA. Ten days later, it reached Britain and Russia. These isotopes have long-term   health   effects. The EPA resumed milk testing in   2012. The isotope levels had lowered due to half-life decay.

Our authorities only tested radiation levels of uranium and   plutonium,   which   are the sources of power creation in nuclear power plants. These nuclear reactor alpha particles would not affect the USA and   stay local.   The Fukushima explosion created rare radioactive cesium and iodine particles with shorter half-lives.

Authorities waited one year before testing these beta isotopes, which allowed radiation levels to decrease. Testing resumed after the radioactive daughters' half-lives diminished. The administration increased acceptable radiation levels in food, water, and soil, which rank among the highest on Earth.

The EPA still monitors the beta radiation isotopes, but only if it sends the test filters to a lab within a specific time limit. In 2011, it took 12 months to report beta radiation fallout.

This incident was not isolated. Hundreds of atomic bomb tests rained fallout over America. These events also went unreported. The public remained unaware of potential health risks. Government agencies failed to provide timely, accurate information. This lack of transparency raises questions about food safety standards. This release also highlights the need for improved monitoring systems.

Nuclear weapons testing in the USA during the 1950s and 1960s released radioactive isotopes, particularly iodine-131, across the country, leading to widespread low-level radiation exposure. While a direct causal link is complex to establish conclusively, evidence suggests that this radiation exposure likely contributed to an increased risk of leukemia, especially in children, during that period and in subsequent years, during the 60s and 70s. I knew at least three occasions where my school classmates died of leukemic.

Due to nuclear fallout, in 1961, Mandan, North Dakota, had eight times higher Strontium-90 concentrations in cow's milk than those from Wisconsin or New York. In 2011, radiation was detected in milk samples from the Big Island of Hawaii following the Fukushima disaster. Elevated levels were found in European milk after the Chornobyl accident in 1986. Contaminated milk was discovered in Utah during 1950s Nevada nuclear testing. High Strontium-90 levels were measured in North Dakota milk in 1958.

Radioactive iodine was found in British milk following the 1957 Windscale fire. In 2011, low levels of radioactive iodine-131 were detected in milk samples from California and Washington, linked to the Fukushima incident. After the Three Mile Island accident in 1979, slightly elevated levels of radioactive iodine were found in local milk supplies. In 2013, cesium-137 was detected in milk from farms near the Fukushima Daiichi plant in Japan. Traces of iodine-131 were found in milk samples across Europe in 2011, believed to be from the Fukushima disaster.

Authorities say the long-term effects of radiation exposure through food remain understudied. Do you believe that? Radiation's impact on agriculture extends beyond immediate contamination. Soil can retain radioactive particles for a long time, affecting crop yields and livestock health. Farmers may face economic hardships due to reduced productivity. Consumer trust in food safety erodes as information surfaces, creating ripple effects throughout the agricultural industry.

The Fukushima incident exposed weaknesses in global disaster response protocols. Radiation release revealed gaps in international cooperation on radiation monitoring. Countries struggled to coordinate efforts and share data, which hampered the ability to assess the full scope of contamination and delayed the implementation of protective measures.

The public health implications of long-term radiation exposure remain debated. Some experts argue for more conservative safety thresholds, while others maintain that current standards provide adequate protection. This disagreement fuels public uncertainty and mistrust. I bet most of you reading this chapter have never even heard of radiosity milk testing.

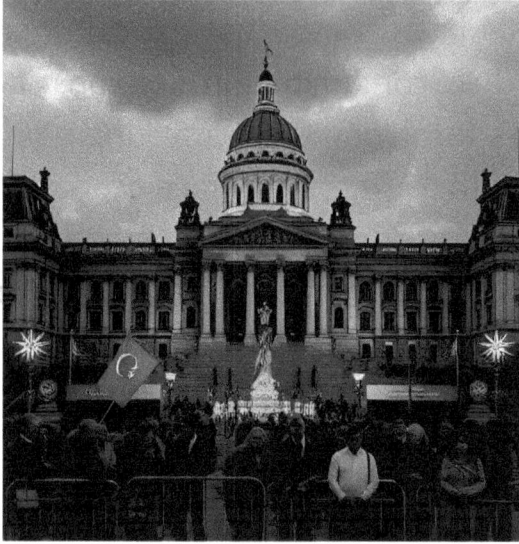

Chapter 18

World Without Compassion: Governments' Disregard For Nuclear Testing Victims

G overnmental disregard affects people with radiation exposure all over the world. Governments mine radioactive minerals and develop nuclear energy without much regard for humanity. When these activities harm people, the authorities downplay, spin, lie, or create false perceptions. Unfortunately, the people suffer and seldom are compensated.

The Soviet Union, with its leader Gorbachev, participated in the atomic race soon after the USA nuclear bomb killed close to 200,000 civilians in Japan. The Soviets rushed into the arms race and tested nuclear weapons in Kazakhstan, an area the size of New Jersey. The Soviets conducted tests near small towns, called villages, some only 20 miles from the perimeter of the designated site called The Polygon.

Soviet nuclear scientists utilized remote test sites for conducting nuclear weapons tests and experiments on humans in nearby villages. In a chilling directive, Gorbachev ordered the execution of scientists and atomic detonation crews if bombs failed to explode. The scientists strategically chose windy days for aboveground bomb tests, allowing radioactive fallout to reach downwind villages. Following these tests, government employees visited the affected villages to observe and document the illnesses sustained by the indigenous population.

This dark chapter of Soviet nuclear testing bears a disturbing resemblance to the Nazi scientists' human experiments discussed earlier in this book. Despite the world's awareness of such atrocities after World War II,

Soviet testing practices continued to disregard human life in the relentless pursuit of nuclear capabilities.

This test site is called the Semipalatinsk Test Site, also known as "The Polygon," the primary location for Soviet nuclear weapons testing from 1949 to 1989. Located in northeastern Kazakhstan, this vast 7,200 square mile area had 456 nuclear tests denoted over four decades. Over these 40 years, the Soviet Union conducted 340 underground and 116 atmospheric tests. The first Soviet atomic bomb was tested at this location on August 29, 1949, marking the beginning of the Soviet nuclear program.

The Soviets employed propaganda in villages surrounding nuclear test sites to bolster their image as a superpower and instill national pride. They convinced locals that their government was benevolent while simultaneously cultivating fear of American aggression, drawing parallels to the atomic bombings in Japan. These tactics mirrored those used by the US government to influence American public opinion. On detonation days, the Soviet government instructed villagers to watch mushroom cloud explosions, unknowingly exposing them to radioactive fallout.

Following these tests, dust and particles rained onto the villagers, their homes, and gardens. People living downstream from nuclear tests experienced sickness, leukemia, and death. The devastating effects became increasingly apparent as residents witnessed the destruction of their families, property, cattle, food sources, and businesses. Gradually, the people began to realize that these weapons were causing immense harm to their communities and way of life.

In a particularly horrific incident, scientists bused 30 children to a nuclear test site to witness a detonation, resulting in the deaths of all 30 children shortly after. The reckless disregard for human life extended to allowing people to swim in radioactive bomb craters. The contamination spread far beyond the test sites, with radioactive soil, air, and water polluting streams and rivers throughout Kazakhstan and Russia. This toxic runoff eventually reached the Arctic Ocean, spreading westward and affecting a vast area.

The consequences for nearby towns were devastating. Residents suffered from severe illnesses, deaths, tumors, and facial disfigurements due to radiation exposure. The Soviet government, in an attempt to conceal these atrocities, censored the affected villagers, threatening punishment for those who spoke about their experiences. The long-term impact of these tests is staggering, with an estimated 1.5 million people expected to be exposed to nuclear weapons fallout over the next four decades, perpetuating a legacy of suffering and environmental destruction.

Radiation from nuclear tests permeated the environment, contaminating soil, air, water, food, and milk. Cows consumed tainted grass, passing radioactive particles to humans through milk consumption. This radiation entered people's bodies, altering DNA and affecting current and future generations. The health consequences were severe, with cancer rates 40% higher than the rest of the country. Approximately 37,000 lung cancers, 31,000 breast cancers, and 23,000 stomach cancers were documented. Nearby towns experienced severe illnesses, deaths, tumors, and facial disfigurements. Today, scientists can observe numerous completely deformed fetuses preserved in jars, which show the lasting effects of radiation exposure.

The impact on life expectancy in these villages was devastating. The average lifespan plummeted to 58 years, with half the population dying before age 63, coinciding with the pension age. Consequently, most villagers never lived long enough to receive a pension check. Economic desperation led many unemployed villagers to collect and sell radioactive metal from test sites at discounted prices. This contaminated metal was often shipped to China for recycling, raising concerns about its potential use in various products and structures. The radioactive scrap metal, with a half-life of 3,000 years, could be present in cars, buildings, materials, homes, and other products, including steel imported by the USA for construction purposes.

The long-term consequences of these nuclear tests continue to affect subsequent generations. Many children in these areas develop mental illnesses, and suicide rates remain high. The Soviet government's response to this tragedy was woefully inadequate. The only compensation offered was a one-time payment of $250, limited to those born before 1969. This meager attempt at reparations did little to address the ongoing suffering and generational trauma experienced by the affected communities.

People started protesting soon after the Semipalatinsk Test Site was closed on August 29, 1991. The closure was mainly due to the efforts of the Nevada-Semipalatinsk Movement, led by Kazakh poet Olzhas Suleimenov. Since its closure, Semipalatinsk has become one of the world's most thoroughly researched atomic testing sites. From 1996 to 2012, a secret joint operation involving Kazakh, Russian, and American nuclear scientists secured leftover plutonium found in the region's mountain tunnels. Today, many nuclear test site zones remain off-limits due to residual contamination.

The United States is no different than other countries when it comes to lies and not compensating those who are made ill by radiation exposures from uranium mining. The Navajo Nation spans 27,000 square miles in the southwestern United States. This uranium-rich region has led to extensive mining activities, which have caused environmental and health havoc for the local population.

Many homes in the Navajo Nation are built using uranium mill tailings waste materials, contributing to elevated indoor radon levels. Combined with uranium-rich soil, this practice produces high radon concentrations in residences, backfill, foundations, and concrete. Residents face a double threat: radiation from uranium, which has a half-life exceeding 2000 years, and radon gas, the second leading cause of lung cancer in the USA.

The severity of the situation in the Navajo Nation is alarming, with some residents unable to occupy the ground floors of their homes due to dangerously high radon concentrations. The entire region suffers from elevated radiation levels from natural sources and abandoned uranium mines (AUMs). Between 1944 and 1986, the extraction of four million tons of uranium left behind over 500 AUMs, scattering radioactive tailings, debris, tools, and metal across numerous locations. This widespread contamination has resulted in a surge of lung cancer, leukemia, and other radiation-related illnesses. Studies have revealed that uranium exposure caused hundreds of premature deaths and thousands of diseases among the Navajo people.

Tragically, the Navajo people were never informed about the risks of contamination or advised to evacuate their homes. The government's failure to compensate affected individuals has left many without access to proper healthcare or financial support for their radiation-induced illnesses. This negligence extends beyond immediate health impacts, as uranium exposure damages DNA, affecting future generations. The US government's refusal to acknowledge and address these issues raises serious concerns about transparency and accountability. As we consider this tragic situation, it prompts unsettling questions: What hidden dangers might exist in our backyards? Would authorities warn us if our homes or neighborhoods faced similar threats?

The Yunkom Mine, located near Yenakiieve in Ukraine's Donetsk region, has a dark history intertwined with uranium mining and nuclear experimentation. Originally a coal mine, it became part of the Soviet atomic program. On September 16, 1979, Soviet authorities detonated a 0.2-0.3 kiloton nuclear device 903 meters below the surface, aiming to release trapped methane and reduce mining accidents. This controversial explosion created a glass-lined cavity and a surrounding fractured zone, both contaminated with radionuclides. Mining operations continued until 2002, when the mine closed due to unprofitability.

The mine's closure didn't end its environmental impact. Radioactive contamination spreads throughout the area, affecting soil, water, and building materials. The entire city of Yenakiieve now faces elevated radiation levels, with Geiger counters detecting abnormal readings in the whole town and surrounding areas. Radiation has permeated the soil, backfill, and concrete used in home construction. Many multi-story buildings have uninhabitable ground floors due to high radon levels emanating from radioactive foundations and backfill.

In the documentary "Embittered City," a second-floor apartment dweller with leukemia reported that all his neighbors on floors 2 and 3 had various cancers, including lung, breast, cervix, thorax, stomach, and skin cancers. She stated that many of her neighbors will die because they dont have money for treatment because of no government compensation. Another interviewee said over 10 million radioactive tons of mining scrap metal were dug up and sold to other countries for re-cycling. This interviewee stated that even the city's po-lice chief had a scrap metal business. This incident is not isolated; over 4000 documented radioactive scrap recycling events have occurred worldwide. One must wonder if everyday items like metal table legs, building materials, or certain car parts may be radioactive, po-tentially affecting our lives without our knowledge.

MARKO VOVK

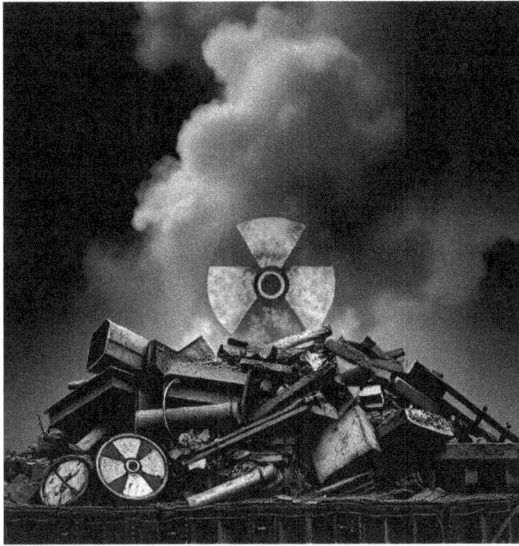

Chapter 19

Radioactive Scrap In Our Everyday Lives

We have discussed radioactive pollution, dumps, leaks, explosions, releases, lies, spins, accidents, and radiation-contaminated sites. Now, let's discuss something nobody is talking about. What if your home or car is becoming the new radiation-contaminated site? Today, scrap metal is collected and recycled. This is a huge business, and China is one of the most prominent scrap collectors.

China is one of the world's lowest virtual water exporters. Depending on the type of steel, it can take up to 66,000 gallons of H2O to produce one ton of metal. Mining, smelting, transportation, and melting all use up water resources. However, according to my research, only a fraction of this water is needed when recycling old cars, say 1,000 gallons. It's funny how this information is not available.

So, the USA uses water to make steel, and China uses a fraction of water to melt and recycle the scrap into new products. So, warm water radiates scrap metal recycling and becomes radioactive. So now, the scrapers, the recyclers, and the water used are contaminated with radiation. Who is wagging the dog here? All over the world, people collect radioactive metals, debris, hospital equipment, bomb-making steel, bomb testing remnants, and mining metal, along with garbage—all of it is radioactive.

Some of this is buried, some in caves, some in water, and some just lying around. Millions of tons of steel and other metals are contained worldwide. Radioactive materials cannot be sensed, seen, or detected without using a calibrated Geiger counter, but most scrappers

NUCLEAR EXTINCTION EVENT IS KILLING OUR FAMILIES

and recyclers don't have these necessary detection devices.

Furthermore, these colorless, odorless, and tasteless radioactive elements or isotopes cannot be visually detected, but they can make people sick and cause death. If you were handed a spent nuclear power plant fuel rod, you would be dead soon. Just being near a spent nuclear power plant fuel rod would result in severe and rapid health consequences due to intense radiation exposure. You would likely experience acute radiation syndrome (ARS) within minutes to hours, with initial symptoms including nausea, vomiting, dizziness, and weakness.

The radiation dose from direct contact would far exceed the threshold for severe ARS, causing extensive and likely irreparable damage to DNA and dividing cells. Without immediate and intensive medical intervention, death would likely occur within hours to days due to rapid deterioration of vital organ systems, including the cardiovascular and central nervous systems.

If you somehow survived the initial exposure, you would face a high risk of developing cancer, leukemia, as well as other long-term health issues such as cardiovascular disease and cataracts. It's essential to understand handling spent nuclear fuel is hazardous and should only be done by trained professionals using specialized equipment and extensive safety measures.

Spent fuel remains radioactive and dangerous for thousands of years after being removed from a nuclear reactor, making any direct contact potentially fatal. Spent fuel rods are extreme, but what about metal like shovels used for uranium mining? What about train carts delivering uranium ore from mines? What about recycled steel? Is it coming from China or anything else that may come into contact with a radioactive substance? Anything that is in contact also becomes radioactive.

Based on data from various sources, over 4,075 confirmed incidents involving radioactive material were mishandled, lost, or disposed of globally between 1993 and 2023. This includes cases where nuclear materials entered the scrap metal recycling chain and other unauthorized activities involving radioactive sources. The IAEA Incident and Trafficking Database (ITDB) has documented hundreds of incidents, averaging 131 per year over the last decade. However, many cases go unreported, suggesting the number could be higher.

In the book, we mentioned the following two sites: The Polygon, Kazakhstan: After the collapse of the Soviet Union, scrap metal from the nuclear testing site was scavenged and sold to China, which recycled it and spread the radioactive contamination.

The Yunkom Mine, Ukraine, which is now an abandoned mine and was the site of a 1979 underground nuclear explosion, had infrastructure sold as scrap metal. The locals and city police chief scrapped and recycled these radioactive metals. These are just a few of the 4000-plus documented radioactive scrap steel collections world-wide.

Vicente Sotelo Alardín and Ricardo Hernández collected the radioactive material sent to steel foundries in Chihuahua and the USA. The contaminated products were distributed across 17 Mexican states and several US cities, exposing 4,000 people to radiation. The Goiânia accident in Brazil 1987 involved a cesium-137 radiotherapy source dismantled by scavengers. Local scrap dealers collected and distributed the material, causing widespread contamination throughout Goiânia. The incident resulted in four deaths and 249 cases of radiation exposure, with over 112,000 people being examined for potential contamination.

In 1998, the Acerinox incident in Spain occurred when a cesium-137 source was melted in a steel factory in Los Barrios. The Acerinox plant processed radioactive isotopes refuse, creating a cloud across Europe. While immediate health impacts were minimal, the incident cost $26 million in cleanup and lost production, affecting various steel products. Istanbul, Turkey, experienced a radioactive scrap incident in 1998-1999 when two cobalt-60 sources were sold as scrap metal. Two brothers, local collectors, obtained the sources from a warehouse. The contaminated materials were processed in a scrapyard and smelting factory outside Istanbul, leading to 18 hospitalizations for radiation exposure.

In 2000, local scrap metal collectors dismantled a cobalt-60 source from a teletherapy unit in Samut Prakan, Thailand. Radioactive ferrous products were taken to a scrapyard in Samut Prakan, resulting in three deaths and ten hospitalizations due to radiation exposure. The Mayapuri incident in India 2010 involved a cobalt-60 source disposed of as scrap metal in New Delhi. Local scrap dealers collected and distributed the material, causing one death and eight injuries.

In 2014, a worker from Tianjin Hongdi Engineering Inspection Development Co. in Nanjing, China, handled a piece of radioactive iridium-192 for hours before discarding it. This triggered a large-scale search operation, resulting in six people diagnosed with health problems and one death. Shaanxi Province, China, experienced a radioactive contamination event 2009 when Xingbao Steel and Iron Company Ltd. melted a cesium-137 source with scrap metal. The contaminated steel products were processed at the No. 6 smelter at Xingbao's factory, causing radioactive slag contamination in backfill or other applications.

In Ohio and Pennsylvania, USA 2016, radium-226-contaminated scrap was shredded and shipped to multiple facilities. PSC Metals in Canton and Massillon, Ohio, detected high radiation levels in the processed materials. Ayutthaya Province, Thailand, faced a potential radioactive incident 2008 when a cesium-137 source was found among scrap metal at a local scrapyard. The material was destined for Chow Steel Industries in Prachin Buri Province. Early detection prevents radiation leakage and potential exposure if you believe it.

In 2008, a recycling factory in Chachoengsao Province, Thailand, triggered alarms when scrap containing radium-226 from an unlicensed lightning preventer was detected. Authorities believe that this contaminated material was sourced from a local scrapyard before being sent to Chow Steel Industries Public Co. Ltd. In a separate incident in 1996, a worker in Jilin, China, suffered severe localized radiation injuries after unknowingly handling an iridium-192 source for about 15 minutes.

The Yanango incident in Peru in 1999 involved a welder who carried an iridium-192 source in his pocket for hours and brought it home. The worker was exposed, requiring amputation, and his family was also affected. In 1999, a cobalt-60 radiotherapy unit sold as scrap caused acute radiation sickness in a family in Henan Province, China. A waste disposal company handled the radioactive material, which ended up in the family's home.

In 1999, Kingisepp, Russia, experienced a tragic incident when scrap thieves stole a radioisotope core from a lighthouse. All three individuals involved died from radiation exposure. In 2003, thieves dismantled radio-thermal generators at lighthouses in Kola Harbor, Russia, seeking to steal metal for scrap. Unshielded strontium-90 sources were recovered nearby. No survivors were identified among the perpetrators.

These above examples represent only a tiny fraction of the documented 4,000 plus incidents; countless more go unreported. It won't be long before we need portable Geiger counties when shopping for cars, appliances, and food. It won't be long before we must test everything in our homes to ensure our family's safety. If we fail to take these precautions, we may expose ourselves and our families to dangerous radiation. The risk of sleeping on a radioactive box bed spring or using

contaminated household items like forks could cause
cancer.

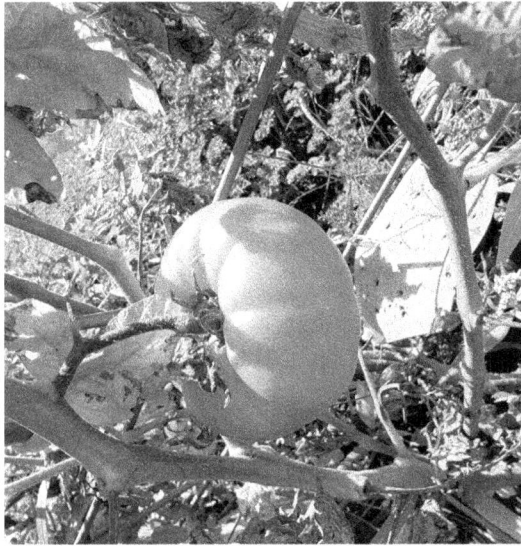

Chapter 20

We Now Eat Radioactive Food

R adioactivity, discovered in 1896, has revolution-
ized our understanding of food safety, transform-
ing from an unknown phenomenon to a powerful tool
in modern food science. Today, scientists harness radiation's dual nature, using techniques like food irradiation to eliminate harmful microorganisms and extend shelf life, while simultaneously dealing with the
risks of radioactive food and water contamination. Ra-

dioactivity's omnipresence in our environment extends from the Earth's crust to the atmosphere. We receive some radiation from natural sources like radon gas from the ground, cosmic rays from the sun, and even trace amounts in foods such as nuts and bananas. While we cannot eliminate these natural sources, we face additional, unnatural radiation exposure from contaminated water and food.

Eighty years ago, our food and water supplies were largely free from radioactive contamination, as humanity had not yet unleashed the power of the atom through nuclear weapons, mining, or power generation. This era of relative radiological purity in our environment came to an abrupt end on July 16, 1945, when the United States detonated the world's first nuclear weapon in the New Mexican desert as part of the Trinity test. This pivotal moment marked the beginning of widespread radioactive contamination of our food and water resources. The explosion dispersed radioactive fallout over an area of more than 1,100 square miles, with some debris reaching as far north as Canada. Hundreds of more nuclear tests conducted between 1945 and 1962 in New Mexico and Nevada further exacerbated this contamination, affecting 46 of the 48 contiguous United States, as well as parts of Canada and Mexico. The spread of radioactive materials from these tests not only contaminated soil and water sources but also entered the food chain through vegetation and livestock.

The nuclear arms race, initiated by the United States in 1945, quickly engulfed other world powers, leading to widespread global radioactive contamination. Russia, China, England, and France join the race, conducting their own nuclear tests and contributing to the spread of radioactive materials. These nations detonate hundred's of nuclear bombs in various locations, from remote deserts to Pacific Atolls, dispersing radioactive fallout across the world. The contamination knows no borders, affecting all food chains, all water sources, and all ecosystems worldwide. Atmospheric and underground tests by these countries release radioactive particles that enter the global environment, impacting lands far from the test sites. This international nuclear activity fundamentally altering of our planet, leaving a lasting legacy of contamination of everything of the surface earth.

In the United States, areas downwind of the Nevada Test Site, including parts of Utah, Nevada, and Arizona, still show high levels of radioactive elements in soil and groundwater. This contamination affects local agriculture, with crops grown in these area absorbing radionuclides like strontium-90 and cesium-137. Milk from cows grazing on contaminated pastures in these regions contains higher levels of radioactive iodine-131, posing a particular risk to children's thyroid.

Globally, the effects of nuclear testing on food and water supplies extend far beyond test sites. In Kazakhstan, the area surrounding the former Semipalatinsk Test Site continues to have elevated levels of radioactivity in soil and water sources. Local produce and livestock from this region contained higher concentrations of radionuclides increasing cancer. Similarly, in the Pacific, former test sites like the Marshall Islands still deal with contaminated soil and water, irradiating local fisheries and agriculture. Consumption of contaminated foods from these areas lead to increased various cancers, including thyroid, leukemia, and bone cancer, as well as potential developmental issues in children.

Uranium mining and processing have left lots of radioactive contamination in numerous areas across the United States. In the Navajo Nation, spanning parts of Arizona, New Mexico, and Utah, abandoned uranium mines have contaminated water sources since the 1950s. The contamination has seeped into groundwater and surface water, affecting drinking water and agricultural irrigation. In Sanders, Arizona, a predominantly Navajo community has been exposed to uranium levels in tap water exceeding many times the legal limit.

The Puerco River basin in New Mexico and Arizona has also been impacted, with radioactive water and sediment released from uranium mining activities contaminating water used by residents and livestock. In the Western United States, over 160,000 abandoned hard rock mines have created chronic exposure conditions for Native American communities. These mines have contaminated soil and water with metal mixtures, including radioactive elements.

The Wind River Reservation in Wyoming, home to the Eastern Shoshone and Northern Arapaho tribes, faces health concerns due to a former uranium mill and its remediated waste pile. In New Mexico, the Homestake Mining Company's uranium mill contaminated groundwater with uranium and selenium, affecting nearby communities for decades. The pollution spread to farmlands through irrigation, contaminating topsoil with elevated levels of radioactive materials. These examples represent only a fraction of the mining areas that have impacted food and water supplies.

In South Africa's Witwatersrand basin, inadequate controls in the uranium mining industry have led to widespread contamination. The region's water sources, including the Wonderfonteinspruit, show alarmingly high levels of radioactivity, with uranium concentrations in sediments reaching up to 10,000 Bq/kg – five times the proposed maximum limit. This contaminated water is used for irrigation, leading to the accumulation of radioactive elements in crops and livestock. Residents in areas such as Carletonville, Westonarea, and Khutsong unknowingly consume contaminated food and water daily.

In Central Asia, the Kyrgyz Republic deals with a legacy of 70 radioactive waste sites, including 36 uranium tailings sites. The Mayluu-Suu site, located just 30 kilometers from Uzbekistan, poses significant environmental problems to the densely populated Ferghana Valley. Local communities rely on contaminated water sources for drinking and agriculture, resulting in the constant ingestion of radioactive materials through their food and water. In Brazil, the Interlagos mill site, which processed radioactive monazite is now affecting local food markets and water supplies.

Canada faces its own problems, with uranium ore contamination at a railhead in its northern regions, impacting indigenous communities who depend on local water sources and traditional foods. Countless other locations, from abandoned mines in the western United States to former nuclear facilities in Europe and Asia, continue to cause havoc on humans. In most of these areas, people unknowingly consume contaminated food and water daily, as radioactive materials continue to enter the food chain through contaminated soil and water used in agriculture and livestock farming.

The global spread of radioactive contamination resembles an unrelenting snowstorm, blanketing the planet with invisible, persistent particles. This radioactive "snow" infiltrates every aspect of our environment - soil, trees, food, animals, insects, and water. Unlike real snow, these particles endure for thousands of years, their presence an unyielding legacy of human nuclear activities. The initial fallout from nuclear testing and uranium mining represents just the first layer of this contamination. As we enter a new era of nuclear power, with the construction of 500 nuclear plants worldwide, we face the prospect of even more potent "storms." These new sources of contamination will add fresh layers to the earth's existing radioactive blanket,

Nuclear power plant incidents, from minor releases to catastrophic meltdowns, augment the global food and water radioactive contamination crisis. Thousands of leaks and releases, often unreported, continuously add to the environmental burden. Each incident contaminates soil and water, setting off a domino effect that impacts drinking water, produce, and livestock. Full-scale meltdowns, like those we've witnessed and will likely see again, unleash unprecedented levels of radioactive material into the environment. These events devastate ecosystems, rendering vast areas uninhabitable and contaminating food and water supplies for generations.

he Fukushima meltdown exemplifies the far-reaching consequences of nuclear disasters. Japan dumped over 10 million radioactive one-ton cleanup bags at thousands of sites, many now leaking, while thyroid cancer rates soar. For a decade, 55 countries banned Japanese food imports, shifting the burden of contaminated produce to nations like the USA and Canada. This crisis shows a pervasive issue: the proximity of nuclear facilities to agricultural areas, increasing the risk of widespread food contamination. The health impact is huge, with Canada's medical care system buckling under the strain. Patients sometimes face up to six-month waits for doctor appointments or CAT scans, a situation potentially linked to long-term exposure to low-level radiation through food and water.

The global contamination of oceans and waterways with radioactive waste is a widespread and ongoing issue involving numerous nations. The United States has dumped tens of thousands of 55-gallon radioactive drums into the oceans, while Russia burns radioactive forests and sinks nuclear submarines. Other countries continue to dump waste into rivers, oceans, and aquifers. This contamination enters the marine food chain, accumulating in fish and seafood consumed worldwide.

As people eat contaminated seafood, radioactive particles build up in their bodies over time. Japan's current release of radioactive water from the Fukushima Daiichi nuclear power plant into the Pacific Ocean is causing immediate ecological impacts. This discharge affects marine life, harming starfish, sea urchins, and West Coast tide pools. Radionuclides enter the marine food chain through phytoplankton and bioaccumulate up to larger organisms. It's also linked to fish, bird, and animal die-offs along affected coastlines. The contamination spreads through ocean currents, affecting fish stocks and seafood far beyond Japan's shores. Consumers worldwide unknowingly ingest these contaminated fish and shellfish, leading to a gradual accumulation of radioactive materials in their bodies.

Simultaneously, contaminated water sources used for irrigation introduce these radioactive elements into crops and livestock. As a result, people consume contaminated food and water daily, with the radioactive burden in their bodies increasing over time. This accumulation will contribute to increased cancer rates and other radiation-related illnesses in affected populations.

The accumulation of radioactive contamination resembles an unrelenting series of snowstorms, each layer adding to the previous one. This "snow" never melts, persisting for thousands of years due to the long half-lives of many isotopes. Our food and water supplies bear the brunt of this contamination, with each new incident adding to the existing burden. Crops absorb radioactive elements from contaminated soil, while livestock consume these crops and contaminated water.

As the "dose" of radiation in our environment increases, we approach a critical threshold. Like a heroin addict facing increasingly potent doses, we risk "overdosing" on accumulated radiation.

 In the United States, the occupational exposure limit is set at 50 mSv per year for workers. The European Union, on the other hand, has a limit of 20 mSv per year for workers, averaged over 5 years. Even though people are the same everywhere, these limits differ due to various reasons. The EU tends to take a more cautious approach to safety, while historical factors have led to each region developing its rules separately over time. Public opinion also plays a role, with some EU countries implementing even stricter limits due to public concerns. For example, Belgium limits exposure in homes to 20-40% of the EU recommendation.

Radiation monitoring in imported food is alarmingly inconsistent. While countries set limits for radionuclides, enforcement varies widely. U.S. Customs uses radiation detection equipment, but not all ports have equal capabilities. Testing methods require expensive equipment and specialized training, making comprehensive screening very difficult. The FDA's approach has changed over time, recently relaxing measures for Japanese radioactive imports. This inconsistency in testing procedures leaves consumers in the dark about radiation levels in their food and water. The true extent of radioactive contamination in our food supply remains uncertain and unknown.

The global spread of radioactive contamination is relentless, with spent nuclear fuel rods, decommissioned power plants, accidents, and military applications all contributing to this pervasive issue. This radioactive "snowfall" continues to accumulates and infiltrate our environment, affecting soil, water, and food supplies worldwide. Spent fuel rods and decommissioning waste create long-term storage problems, while depleted uranium munitions contaminate conflict zones.

These sources introduce more and more radioactive materials into our ecosystems, where they persist for thousands of years. As this contamination accumulates, it inevitably enters our food chain and water supplies.

Crops absorb radioactive particles from contaminated soil, while livestock consume these crops and drink from tainted water sources. Seafood becomes more contaminated as radionuclides make their way into rivers and oceans.

This cycle ensures a constant influx of radioactive materials into our diet. We unknowingly consume these radioactive isotopes daily, leading to a gradual buildup of radiation in our bodies. If this trend continues unchecked, we risk approaching a critical threshold – a radiation "overdose" on a global scale. This will lead to increased rates of cancer, genetic mutations, and other radiation-related illness across populations.

The nuclear industry's tight control over radiation information in our food supply is alarming. Despite official claims of low, natural levels, the reality may be far more concerning. Generic responses about trace amounts of potassium-40 or carbon-14 in bananas or Brazil nuts or radiation from the sun or flying in jets mask a darker truth. As man-made, accidental, or discarded radiation continues to accumulate in our environment like unmelting snow, the full extent of contamination remains obscured.

The suppression of data and difficulty in accessing accurate information should raise red flags for the entire planet. To uncover the truth, individuals need to take matters into their own hands. Purchasing personal radiation detection equipment, while still legal and available, could become necessity for testing everyday items like salmon, rice, and bottled water at the supermarket. As regulations tighten, these tools may become harder to obtain.

The ongoing buildup of radioactive elements in our food chain resembles an intensifying addiction. Without transparency and accurate data, we risk unknowingly consuming increasingly potent doses of radiation, approaching a critical threshold for public health. It won't be long become we start to wear radiation detections dosomenterts.

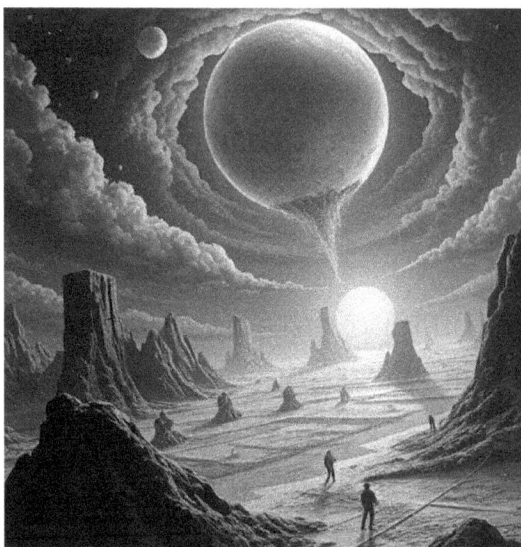

Chapter 21

The Next Extinction Event

E arth has experienced five major extinction events throughout its history, each leaving an indelible mark on its biodiversity. These cataclysmic occurrences have reshaped life on Earth multiple times, paving the way for new species to evolve and thrive in the aftermath.

The Ordovician-Silurian extinction, which occurred approximately 445 million years ago, is an example of nature's power to reshape the planet. Triggered by global cooling, this event decimated 85% of marine species and fundamentally altered the composition of Earth's oceans.

The Permian-Triassic extinction, often called the "Great Dying," occurred 252 million years ago and proved even more devastating. Volcanic eruptions on an unprecedented scale lead to global warming, ultimately eliminating 96% of all species. This event represents the closest life on Earth has come to destruction.

The Cretaceous-Paleogene extinction, which occurred 66 million years ago, is perhaps the most well-known of these events due to its role in ending the dinosaurs' reign. An asteroid impact of immense proportions triggered worldwide cooling and caused widespread ecosystem collapse. The aftermath of this event saw the rise of mammals as the dominant land vertebrates, setting the stage for the eventual emergence of humans.

While catastrophic, these extinction events have played a massive role in shaping the diversity of life we see today, creating opportunities for surviving species to adapt and evolve and filling newly vacant ecological niches. As we look to the future, scientists propose various scenarios for potential extinction events that could reshape life on Earth once again, including asteroid impacts, supervolcano eruptions, cosmic radiation, human-induced climate change, polar shifts, global pandemics, and even more speculative threats like artificial intelligence or alien invasions.

The scientists and people of this planet need to think seriously about the newest extinction event occurring right now. For the last eighty years, this event has been killing millions of people and destroying our planet. Unearthing radioactive minerals and creating dangerous isotopes by manipulating them triggers the next extinction event.

The telltale signs are evident, and they gave us hints even in the early stages when man discovered how to use these radioactive minerals. Man should have seen this when The Radium Girls tragedy exposed the dangers of these elements. Factory workers who painted watch dials with radium-laced paint suffered horrific deaths from radiation poisoning.

Despite the Radium Girls incident, humans continued to exploit radioactive materials. The development of atomic bombs ignored Einstein's warnings about their destructive potential. Nuclear weapons testing contaminated vast areas of land, water, and atmosphere with long-lasting radioactive fallout. These contaminated areas are getting larger and larger, and man can no longer inhabit them.

After we created thousands of atomic weapons, enough to blow up the entire planet 4 times, along with many accidents and many lost weapons under water and ice, we decided to use these radioactive elements and isotopes to create energy. Before we built 500 nuclear reactors, we had the first atomic reactor meltdown in 1959 at Santa Susana Field Laboratory. This event released nuclear material into the environment, making people sick, and yet, atomic power expansion continued.

Even after many more accidents that killed many people and made millions sick, along with land contamination, making it uninhabitable, we had more accidents like Three Mile Island, Chornobyl, and Fukushima, which caused worldwide devastation. Even after these, we continued to implement the use of these radioactive elements.

These nuclear power plants are being abandoned, becoming outdated, decommissioned, leaking, melting, and making people sick who live in these areas or downstream. Some nuclear reactors are not scheduled to be demolished for 100 years because no funds exist to do the work. Still today, these power plants have hundreds of thousands of radioactive spent fuel rods that nobody knows what to do with, and nobody wants them; despite this, they keep mining, enriching, and making new ones. This radiation is entering our lakes, rivers, oceans, and wells. It contaminates the land and trees and will continue for hundreds of thousands of years. Some of these radioactive elements and isotopes have half-lives of millions of years.

We even recycled some of these radioactive isotopes and waste and put them into munitions. Depleted uranium, a byproduct of nuclear fuel production, found its way into munitions. These weapons spread radioactive dust across battlefields worldwide. We now have many countries riddled with these radioactive bullets, killing insects, plants, animals, and children who find them and play with them. Today, because of these radioactive bullets, we now have increased congenital disabilities and declining fertility rates in affected areas, suggesting long-term health consequences for exposed populations.

What's worse is we dumped hundreds of thousands of barrels of radioactive waste into our oceans all over the world. Most of these are rusted and have become part of our ocean bottoms. We eat the radioactive fish and put it in our food. We sink radioactive submarines, some with people in them, and they lay rotting and leaking at the bottom of our ocean. Instead of our governments decreasing our exposure limits, we increase them, giving the illusion that everything is fine.

We even blow up underground rock to extract gas and oil, releasing radioactive elements into the water, air, and waste. Fracking waste containing radiological material has been repurposed as road de-icing agents. These substances are sprayed on roads to melt snow and ice, and the de-icers run off the streets. This practice introduces radiation into water systems, affecting wildlife and ecosystems. Studies show that road runoff causes endocrine disruption in amphibians and insect die-offs.

The insanity does not stop many countries from having nuclear weapons and threatening to use them in wars, proxy wars, or religious wars. This nuclear proliferation has placed world-ending weapons in multiple countries that should not have them. What if an accident occurs, or the wrong person gets hold of them? We have already had accidents where plane collisions, fires, or other incidents dropped nuclear weapons to the ground. These accidents happened in France, Greenland, and even the US. The 1961 Goldsboro B-52 crash nearly detonated a nuclear bomb on US soil. Such incidents highlight the risks of accidental nuclear war or terrorist acquisition of nuclear materials.

The worst part is that our leaders and governments lie, spin, or deflect reality. Today, as you read this, Japan has millions of 1-ton radioactive waste bags from the Fukushima nuclear meltdown cleanup that are stored all over the country, and many are already leaking. They know this because the throat cancers and problems now in Japan are off the charts. Even after one decade of only one nuclear power plant meltdown, the Pacific Ocean continues to become contaminated, and the starfish and sea urchins are dying along with fish, birds, and mammal die-offs. This is only one nuclear power plant; they still need billions to clean up, and it has already been a decade.

We even use these radioactive isotopes in our medical and dental industries. How many dental X-rays do you need? We irradiate our cancers and drink radioactive substances for CT scans. Do you ever wonder why the X-ray technicians stand outside the room and why you're getting irradiated?

Why can't we see why cancer rates are skyrocketing globally? In 2024, over 2 million new cancer cases are expected in the United States alone. This represents 5,500 new diagnoses every day. The incidence is increasing for 6 of the top 10 most common cancers.

Why can't we see birth rates plummeting worldwide, with many developed nations facing population decreases? Environmental toxins, including radiation exposure, may contribute to reduced fertility. Some studies suggest sperm counts have dropped by over 50% in Western countries since the 1970s.

Why can't we see nuclear accidents, leaks, and failures pose a grave threat to our planet's future? Widespread radioactive contamination will devastate ecosystems, disrupt food webs, and cause irreversible genetic damage across generations. As nuclear winter scenarios predict severe global cooling, agricultural collapse will follow, leading to widespread famine. Long-lived radioactive isotopes will persist in the environment for millennia, contaminating water resources and rendering vast areas uninhabitable for countless species, including humans.

The ripple effects of nuclear disasters extend far beyond immediate environmental impacts. Chronic radiation exposure causes cumulative genetic damage, altering the course of evolution for countless species. These effects, combined with existing environmental stressors like extreme weather and habitat loss, create a perfect storm of ecological devastation.

Major nuclear disasters have theological, economic, and social impacts, causing societal collapse and indirectly accelerating global ecosystem breakdown. As these factors converge and intensify, they push our planet towards a tipping point, setting the stage for a catastrophic extinction event.

Food and water supplies face ongoing contamination risks, as evidenced by the Fukushima nuclear disaster, which released radioactive materials into the Pacific Ocean, causing widespread marine death. The continued discharge of tritium-contaminated water raises alarming concerns about long-term impacts on aquatic life and human health.

The future nuclear power plant meltdown looms on the horizon, threatening to devastate another 50,000 square miles of land, rendering more land uninhabitable. This disaster will make millions sick and inflict DNA damage on future generations. We currently have nearly 500 of these ticking time bombs scattered across the globe. It's only a matter of time before another one goes off.

Across the world, millions of spent nuclear fuel rods sit in storage with no clear plan for their disposal. Imagine this: someone carelessly takes one and places it in a shed. Suddenly, eight billion people could unknowingly walk into that shed and touch the rod, leading to all deaths. After killing eight billion, this single spent nuclear rod remains dangerously radioactive for thousands of more years.

Even the metal bedpost in your bedroom, the beams in your house, or the frame of your car may be radioactive due to leaks from refueling operations. You might be getting sick without even realizing it. Consider this: just one pound of plutonium can accidentally irradiate an entire city of 10 million people.

Our media shows us skinny polar bears and tells us it's climate change. Maybe these polar bears have leukemia from all the sunken nuclear submarines under the Arctic, radiated air from radioactive forest fires, radioactive plumes from meltdowns, or from eating radioactively contaminated seals. I bet they never did an autopsy on one of these skinny bears.

Anyone who dismisses this risk or advocates for nuclear energy is turning a blind eye to Earth's new extinction event.

Humanity's reckless use of radioactive materials threatens Earth's future. Will the slow accumulation of radiation trigger the next mass extinction? Or will human shortsightedness lead to a more sudden cataclysm? The clock ticks as radioactive contamination spreads, leaving us to question whether we can change course before it's too late.

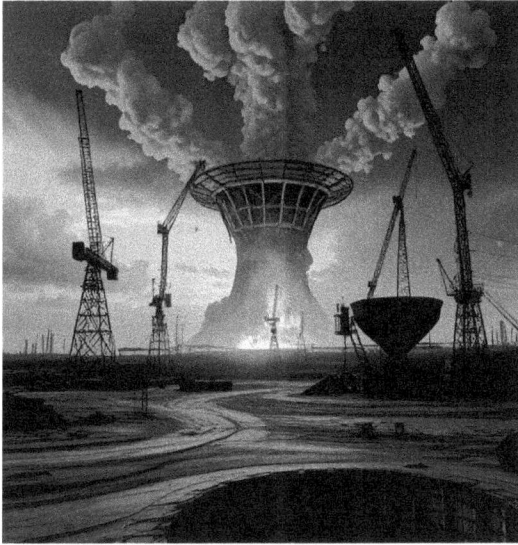

Chapter 22

Appendix A: The Global Nuclear Pollution Players

Radiation exposure plagued human health since the dawn of the atomic age. Nuclear energy, weapons testing, and accidental leaks have left a trail of suffering across generations. Companies like General Electric, Westinghouse, Kodak, and many other government facilities have been implicated in numerous incidents.

The intial players and the Manhattan Project's key corporate contributors were Stone & Webster, Tennessee Eastman (Kodak), Westinghouse Electric, and General Electric. These companies played crucial roles in developing the world's first nuclear weapons.

Stone & Webster, founded in 1889, built the Y-12 electromagnetic separation plant at Oak Ridge during the Manhattan Project. This facility produced enriched uranium for the first atomic bombs. The company significantly contributed to nuclear facility construction throughout the Cold War. Today, Stone & Webster operates as a division of Westinghouse Electric Company, providing engineering services in the nuclear and energy sectors.

Stone & Webster now faces billions in costs for decommissioning nuclear plants it built, including Yankee Rowe, Maine Yankee, Connecticut Yankee, and Millstone. The U.S. government and taxpayers subsidize these efforts through the Nuclear Waste Fund, utility rate increases, and federal loan guarantees. These subsidies address the underestimated original decommissioning costs. The company now manages these complex projects and, in my opinion, might go broke soon with all the regulatory costs that keep amplifying the world's nuclear industry.

Tennessee Eastman (Kodak), founded in 1920 as a Kodak subsidiary, managed the Y-12 plant in Oak Ridge, Tennessee, during the Manhattan Project, training operators for uranium isotope separation. After the project's closure, the company secretly transported uranium-235 to its headquarters in Rochester, New York, storing it beneath its office tower for research and quality control.

Recently, the U.S. government discovered this concealed contamination. Questions arise about the health impacts on building janitors. Kodak was also involved in the production of Agent Orange, which was dumped by aerosol injection from airplanes and covered Vietnam an estimated four times over. Agent Orange was reportedly burned at night to dispose of excess chemicals. The company's activities have been linked to environmental sickness in the Rochester, NY, area, including issues similar to those at Love Canal, where residents near Lake Ontario have reported increased rates of illness and mortality.

Eastman Chemical, now independent from Kodak, is a global specialty materials company. However, it still faces ongoing environmental cleanup efforts, potential health claims, and lawsuits related to its past involvement in the nuclear industry. Thus, it may face significant financial constraints in future years.

Westinghouse Electric Company, founded in 1999, is a subsidiary of the original Westinghouse Electric Corporation's nuclear division. It supplies uranium metal for atomic research and develops pressurized water reactor technology. Cameco and Brookfield Asset Management own Westinghouse. It focuses on nuclear services and advanced designs like the AP1000.

The AP1000 nuclear reactor operates in China, with four units in service and eight under construction. Two AP1000 units at Vogtle Electric Generating Plant in Georgia have entered commercial operation. These are the U.S.'s first nuclear construction projects in over thirty years. When I was a kid, I only touched the stove once.

Westinghouse was criticized for cost overruns at the Vogtle nuclear plant expansion in Georgia, which led to its bankruptcy filing in 2017. The project's final cost reached $36.8 billion, double the initial estimate. Overruns result from design changes, construction delays, and regulatory laws.

Today, Westinghouse decommissions old nuclear plants and develops new small modular reactors. It provides atomic fuel and maintenance services to existing facilities worldwide and supplies uranium fuel mined in Kazakhstan, Canada, and Australia. Resource extraction and mining continue to cause environmental damage through water and soil contamination, air pollution, deforestation, erosion, and biodiversity loss. Local Indigenous people face land dispossession, cultural destruction, health impacts, lack of consent, economic marginalization, and continued violence due to extraction activities on their territories.

General Electric, founded in 1892 in New York, provided electrical equipment and support for Manhattan Project facilities. GE developed nuclear technologies, including reactors and fuel, becoming a major conglomerate in the nuclear industry. The company designed 87 nuclear reactors worldwide, including 35 in the US and 25 in Japan. These designs are similar to the ones that failed at Fukushima, where spent fuel rods were stored above the reactors instead of in separate buildings.

GE faced radioactive contamination issues at several of its facilities across the USA. One of these sites was Nela Park in East Cleveland, Ohio. Although no longer operational, the site remains guarded due to ongoing contamination concerns. The facility produced fluorescent lamps containing radioactive materials, primarily thorium and uranium. Soil and groundwater contamination have been reported, with radium-226 and thorium-232 as the primary contaminants.

GE has implemented containment measures, including a groundwater treatment system, but complete cleanup plans and costs are not publicly available. Reports of illness among former workers and nearby residents have emerged, but specific lawsuit information is limited. In the 1950s, my father, who held two doctorates and was a principal of a teacher's school in Trieste, Italy, was hired by GE as a post-Manhattan Project scientist to work on Nela Computer and design lightbulbs.

While working at the Nela facility, my father became ill and later mysteriously died of leukemia. After he quit, many strange events occurred, including an incident where his truck had all four tires simultaneously blow out, causing him to almost die with multiple broken bones. I believe these incidents were related to the secrecy surrounding the nuclear industry. My father was a victim of this industry, and my family suffered. My mother never knew the truth and was told he was sick from a rare bone disease, despite his seven brothers and sisters living in Slovenia, all living until their 90s while his life was cut in half. Our family never filed lawsuits because we were not informed and ignorant, just like millions worldwide who were and still are being deceived.

Today, GE's nuclear operations continue through GE Hitachi Nuclear Energy, focusing on advanced reactor designs like the BWRX-300 small modular reactor. While no BWRX-300 units have been built yet, several countries have shown interest. The estimated cost per unit is around $1 billion, though this figure may be optimistic. GE faces continued issues in nuclear waste management and decommissioning costs for its existing reactors, with estimates running into hundreds of billions of dollars. The long-term costs and potential health and environmental impacts of these new technologies remain uncertain, as do the decommissioning costs after 40 years of use and potential leaks or new health issues.

Électricité de France (EDF), established in 1946 in Paris, operates 56 nuclear reactors in France. These reactors produce 70% of the country's electricity. EDF disposes of atomic waste at the La Hague reprocessing plant and plans deep geological storage. Some waste leaks have occurred in the past, affecting groundwater and soil.

EDF is concerned about its aging reactors, many of which are approaching their 40-year design lifespan. The company needs billions of dollars for maintenance and life extensions. However, it lacks sufficient funds for decommissioning, estimated at 300 billion euros for the entire fleet. The government may need to intervene.

The Flamanville 3 project, a new EPR reactor, has been delayed for over a decade and has tripled in cost to over 20 billion dollars. The EPR uses uranium oxide fuel enriched up to 4.95% U-235, aiming for higher efficiency and safety than older reactors. EDF struggles with welding issues in critical pipework and regulatory requirements for safety systems. The project has difficulties building new nuclear plants, including complex designs, skilled labor shortages, and stringent safety regulations.

France plans to nationalize EDF, meaning the government will fully own the company. This move aims to fund new projects and ensure energy security. Nationalization may lead to higher electricity prices for consumers. Today, EDF faces criticism for underestimating project costs and timelines and continues to have controversies regarding transparency in reporting safety incidents at its nuclear facilities.

China General Nuclear Power Group operates 24 nuclear units in China and projects in other countries. CGN evolved from earlier state-owned atomic companies, including the Ministry of Nuclear Industry. China conducted 45 nuclear tests at Lop Nor, releasing radioactive isotopes like strontium-90 and cesium-137. The test area covers 39,000 square miles and affects nearby populations with increased cancer rates and congenital disabilities. These lands are highly contained today and will remain so for thousands of years.

CGN's reactors are primarily pressurized water reactors using uranium fuel, with the oldest dating to the 1990s. The French company Framatome built many of these reactors. The US restricts nuclear trade with CGN due to concerns about technology transfer to China's military, limiting CGN's access to US nuclear technology and expertise.

China's most radioactive sites remain undisclosed due to state secrecy. The communist government controls information about nuclear issues, and affected populations often lack recourse for compensation or treatment.

CGN develops small modular and thorium-based molten salt reactors, with several demonstration projects under construction in China. Thorium reactors use thorium-232, which is more abundant than uranium. China plans to build its first commercial thorium reactor by 2030. Though designers claim improved safety features, these reactors can potentially leak radioactive materials. China's handling of radiation-affected populations remains opaque, with limited public information on compensation or treatment programs.

Korea Electric Power Corporation (KEPCO), established in 1898 and headquartered in Naju, operates 24 nuclear reactors in South Korea. For the Barakah Nuclear Power

Plant, KEPCO exported its APR-1400 reactor design to the United Arab Emirates. The company faces issues due to South Korea's shifting energy policies under different administrations. These include financial strain from policy-driven nuclear plant closures and uncertainty in long-term investment planning.

Former President Moon Jae-in's administration pursued a nuclear power phase-out from 2017 to 2022. This policy aimed to reduce nuclear and coal power in favor of renewable energy, citing safety concerns post-Fukushima. President Yoon reversed this policy in 2022, supporting atomic energy expansion. These policy shifts create uncertainty for KEPCO's long-term planning and investments in the nuclear sector. Examples include the halted construction of the Shin Hanul 3 and 4 reactors and the premature closure of the Wolsong 1 reactor.

KEPCO pursues opportunities in small modular reactors (SMRs) and hydrogen production using nuclear power. The company is developing the SMART (System-integrated Modular Advanced Reactor) design. No SMRs are currently operational, but several are in the planning and design phase. The company plans to build four small modular reactors by 2030. These will likely use low-enriched uranium fuel with enrichment levels below 5% U-235.

The South Korean government funds these projects through research grants and public-private partnerships. South Korea's leading nuclear waste storage site is the Gyeongju Low and Intermediate Level Radioactive Waste Disposal Center. It currently stores waste from nuclear power plants, hospitals, and research facilities. It can store 800,000 drums of low- and intermediate-level waste, including contaminated tools, clothing, and resins. High-level waste, primarily spent nuclear fuel, remains in temporary storage at nuclear plant sites, awaiting a permanent solution. As of 2024, South Korea has accumulated approximately 19,000 tons of spent nuclear fuel stored in cooling pools at reactor sites.

Framatome, founded in 1958 and based in Paris, designs and supplies nuclear steam systems, equipment, services, and fuel. The company has constructed over 100 reactors worldwide. Framatome's systems have encountered issues, including welding problems at the Flamanville EPR in France and delays at the Olkiluoto plant in Finland.

The company's EPR (Evolutionary Power Reactor) design uses enriched uranium oxide fuel. Four EPRs are operational globally, with several more planned or under construction. Framatome faces many problems with project delays and cost overruns, particularly with the

EPR design. The Flamanville 3 project in France is over a decade late and three times over budget.

Framatome, through its parent company Orano, manages nuclear waste at the La Hague reprocessing plant in France. This facility stores and reprocesses spent nuclear fuel, which contains high-level radioactive waste, including plutonium, uranium, and fission products. The plant discharges approximately 230 million liters of nuclear waste into the Atlantic Ocean annually, with water samples near the discharge pipe showing radiation levels up to 3,900 times higher than background levels.

High concentrations of dangerous radioisotopes have been detected, including Cesium-137 (22,000 Bq/kg), Cobalt-60 (355 Bq/kg), and Americium-241 (53 Bq/kg). The English Channel near La Hague has cesium-137 concentrations of 8 Bq/m^3, compared to 0.6 Bq/m^3 in the Southern Atlantic.

Krypton-85 levels in the air in La Hague were measured at 93,000 Bq/m^3, compared to the average of 1-2 Bq/m^3. The French government and taxpayers bear a significant portion of the costs for decommissioning and waste management, with the cleanup of the Marcoule site estimated to cost about €6 billion in 2003. Countries with reprocessing contracts at La Hague, including Germany, Belgium, the Netherlands, Switzerland, Spain, and Japan, share some responsibility for the nuclear waste. However, the exact distribution of costs is not specified.

This is a brief list of some of the key players in nuclear pollution who have contributed to millions of deaths and illnesses around the globe since these radioactive substances were unearthed and manipulated. Let's look at more nuclear players who directly and indirectly impact the world's atomic crises.

Orano, founded in 2018, succeeds Areva as a nuclear fuel cycle company operating from France. It provides global uranium mining, conversion, enrichment, reprocessing services, and handling of uranium and plutonium isotopes for atomic power plants. Orano manages nuclear waste at La Hague, discharging radioactive waste materials into the English Channel and affecting marine ecosystems. These discharges harm aquatic life by causing genetic mutations, reducing reproductive success, and disrupting the food chain. The company faces criticism for contamination and financial issues inherited from Areva's past nuclear projects, impacting its operations in the global nuclear market.

Toshiba, established in 1875 in Japan, manufactures nuclear reactors and provides related services worldwide. The company has supplied over 30 nuclear reactors globally, primarily to countries like Japan, the United States, and China. It works with uranium and plutonium isotopes, supplying global components and systems for nuclear power plants. Toshiba doesn't directly manage nuclear waste but contributes to plant decommissioning efforts in Japan and other countries. Specialized government agencies or contracted companies in each country where Toshiba's reactors operate typically handle nuclear waste management. For instance, in Japan, the Nuclear Waste Management Organization (NUMO) is responsible for the disposal of high-level radioactive waste. The company faced financial troubles due to its US nuclear subsidiary Westinghouse's bankruptcy in 2017.

Mitsubishi Heavy Industries, founded in 1884 in Japan, designs and builds nuclear reactors for domestic and international markets. It has supplied over 20 nuclear reactors globally, primarily to countries like Japan and the United States. MHI handles uranium fuel and develops advanced reactor designs, including small modular reactors for various clients worldwide. While MHI has been creating small modular reactor designs, none have been built commercially yet. The company contributes to Japan's nuclear waste management efforts but doesn't operate its disposal sites. In Japan, nuclear waste management is primarily handled by the Nuclear

Waste Management Organization (NUMO). MHI faced complications with the San Onofre nuclear plant shutdown, leading to legal disputes and impacts on future projects.

Hitachi, founded in 1910 in Japan, manufactures nuclear reactors and other equipment for global clients. It has supplied over 20 nuclear reactors globally, primarily to countries like Japan and the United States. Hitachi works with uranium fuel and develops boiling water reactor technology for nuclear power plants worldwide, such as the Advanced Boiling Water Reactor (ABWR) design used in Japan and Taiwan.

Some Hitachi-built reactors, such as those at Fukushima Daiichi, experienced problems during the 2011 disaster. Hitachi contributes to decommissioning projects in Japan but doesn't directly manage nuclear waste disposal sites. The company is involved in decommissioning efforts at Fukushima Daiichi, developing specialized robots and equipment. However, several robots deployed at Fukushima failed due to extremely high radiation levels. For instance, in 2017, a robot designed to inspect the damaged reactor core of Unit 2 had to be abandoned after its camera failed, likely due to radiation exposure exceeding 650 Sieverts per hour. This level would be lethal to humans in seconds. Hitachi withdrew from the UK Wylfa nuclear project in 2020, citing financial concerns, potentially limiting its future role in international atomic development.

Bechtel, founded in 1898 in the USA, provides engineering and construction services for nuclear facilities worldwide. These services include design, construction, and project management for nuclear power plants, waste treatment facilities, and decommissioning projects. It handles various radioactive materials during the construction and decommissioning of nuclear plants and waste management facilities. Bechtel's role typically involves containment and safe handling of these materials, but specialized agencies or plant operators usually manage disposal. Bechtel manages nuclear waste cleanup projects, including work at the Hanford Site and the Waste Isolation Pilot Plant. At Hanford, Bechtel is constructing the Waste Treatment Plant to vitrify radioactive waste. The company has faced criticism for cost overruns and delays in nuclear projects, potentially affecting its future contracts in the industry. For example, the Vogtle nuclear plant project in Georgia, where Bechtel took over construction in 2017, has seen its costs balloon from an initial estimate of $14 billion to over $30 billion, with delays in completion.

Cameco, established in 1988 in Canada, focuses on uranium mining, refining, conversion, and fuel manufacturing. It was formed by merging two Crown corporations: Eldorado Nuclear Limited and Saskatchewan Mining Development Corporation. Cameco produces uranium for nuclear power plants globally, handling various uranium isotopes throughout the fuel cycle. The company's operations include mines in Saskatchewan and Kazakhstan, but historically, uranium mining also occurred at Great Bear Lake in the Northwest Territories. The mining at Great Bear Lake, conducted by Eldorado Gold Mines (a predecessor company), caused significant environmental damage and health issues for local Indigenous workers, leading to what became known as the "widows of Déline" due to high cancer rates among former miners.

Cameco manages waste from uranium mining and processing at its operational sites, impacting surrounding environments and communities. The company employs tailings management facilities and water treatment processes to contain and treat mining waste. Due to low uranium prices in recent years, Cameco suspended operations at some mines, including McArthur River and Rabbit Lake. The low uranium prices were primarily due to oversupply in the market following the Fukushima disaster in 2011, which reduced demand as some countries scaled back their nuclear power programs. Additionally, increased production from Kaza-khstan and other sources contributed to oversupply.

However, recent trends indicate a potential turnaround in the uranium market. According to the latest data, uranium prices have increased since 2023, with spot prices reaching $81.75/lb as of August 8, 2024. This represents a significant increase from previous years, although it's still below the peak prices in early 2024. The company has already begun ramping up production at some sites. McArthur River/Key Lake is expected to produce up to 19 million pounds (100% basis) in 2024, an increase from the previous estimate of 18 million pounds.

Rerenco, founded in 1970 with facilities in the UK, Germany, Netherlands, and USA, provides uranium enrichment services. Enrichment is increasing the concentration of uranium-235 isotopes in uranium, typically from 0.7% found in nature to 3-5% for use in nuclear reactors. It enriches uranium for nuclear fuel, handling uranium-235 and uranium-238 isotopes for clients worldwide, including nuclear power plants in about 15 countries. Urenco operates a Tails Management Facility for depleted uranium storage. Depleted uranium is the byproduct of the enrichment process, containing a lower concentration of U-235 than natural uranium; the environmental impacts at its enrichment sites include

radiation exposure risks and the long-term management of radioactive waste.

Exelon, formed in 2000 in the USA, operates nuclear
power plants across multiple states, including Illinois,
Pennsylvania, New York, and Maryland. Several of its
plants have experienced radioactive leaks, like at Braidwood, Dresden, and Quad Cities in Illinois. It manages
uranium fuel and produces electricity from nuclear reactors, serving many customers. Exelon stores spent
nuclear fuel on-site at its plants, potentially impacting
surrounding areas through thermal pollution and radiation risks. The company has faced criticism for safety
issues and lobbying for atomic subsidies, and it may face
future problems with aging infrastructure and renewable energy competition.

Duke Energy, established in 1904 in the USA, operates
nuclear power plants as part of its energy portfolio in
the Carolinas and Florida. Its atomic facilities include
Oconee, McGuire, and Catawba in the Carolinas and
Crystal River in Florida. Minor tritium leaks have been
reported at some sites, such as Oconee, in 2019. Duke
Energy stores spent nuclear fuel at its plant sites, with
future environmental impacts on nearby water bodies and communities. In 2014, a leak at the Oconee
plant resulted in radioactive groundwater contamination, though it was contained on-site. The company has

faced issues with coal ash contamination, particularly in North Carolina, and nuclear plant closures, potentially affecting its future nuclear operations and waste management strategies.

NuScale Power, founded in 2007 in the USA, develops small modular reactor (SMR) technology. As of 2024, no NuScale SMRs are in commercial operation, but the company has agreements for potential deployments in several countries. It designs reactors using low-enriched uranium fuel, aiming to provide scalable nuclear power solutions globally. NuScale's designs incorporate features for on-site spent fuel storage, potentially reducing waste transportation but raising concerns about distributed storage. These storage facilities could be compromised by extreme weather events or seismic activity, though NuScale claims their design includes robust safety features.

TerraPower, established in 2006 in the USA, focuses on developing advanced nuclear reactor designs, including the Natrium reactor being developed for a demonstration project in Wyoming. It works on traveling wave and molten chloride fast reactor technologies, using uranium and potentially thorium fuels. The traveling wave reactor design aims to use depleted uranium as fuel, theoretically reducing waste, but faces significant technical concerns. The molten chloride fast reactor uses

molten salt as fuel and coolant, potentially offering improved efficiency but presenting challenges to corrosion and materials. TerraPower's designs aim to reduce
nuclear waste production but still require solutions for
long-term waste management, which remains an indus-
try-wide dream.

Some nuclear industry pollution players have emerged
as financial winners, reaping profits from their operations. In contrast, others have faced significant losses
due to project delays, cost overruns, and market constraints. However, the real losers in this atomic saga
are those who walk this planet and the Earth itself.
The environmental contamination from uranium mining, nuclear accidents, and radioactive waste disposal
has left an indelible mark on ecosystems worldwide.
Communities near nuclear facilities often bear the brunt
of health risks, with increased rates of cancer and other
radiation-related illnesses reported in many areas.

The long-term consequences of nuclear activities, including managing dangerous waste for thousands of
years, pose an intergenerational burden. Moreover, taxpayers often underestimate and subsidize the immense
financial costs of nuclear power, diverting resources
from potentially safer and more sustainable energy solutions. As we continue to deal with the legacy of the
atomic age, it becomes increasingly clear that the actu-

al cost of this technology extends far beyond balance sheets, leaving a complex and lasting impact on human health, environmental integrity, and the future of our planet.

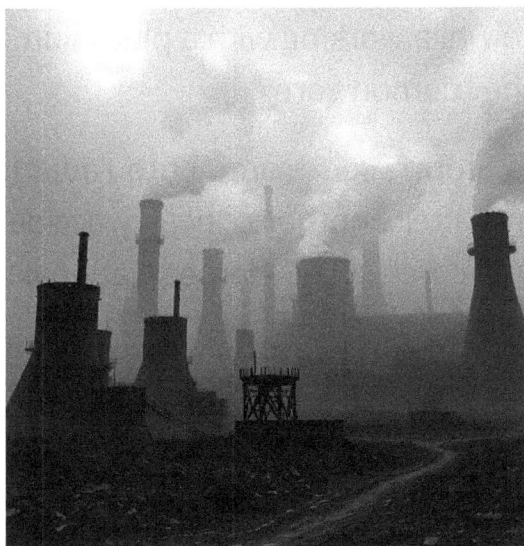

Chapter 23

Appendix B : 100 Nuclear Power Plant And Other Radiant Leaks

N uclear power plants and other major atomic incidents have occurred throughout the history of atomic energy. This list provides only an overview of a handful of documented events. A comprehensive account of all nuclear incidents would require extensive research and a much larger document.

1945: Harry Daghlian was fatally irradiated in a criticality accident at Los Alamos National Laboratory in New Mexico while working with a plutonium bomb core known as the "demon core."

1946: Louis Slotin died from acute radiation poisoning nine days after another criticality accident with the same "demon core" at Los Alamos National Laboratory.

1948: A fire at the Hanford Site in Washington state released radioactive particles over a 200-square-mile area.

1949: A criticality accident occurred at the Los Alamos Scientific Laboratory in New Mexico, exposing one person to a high radiation dose.

1950: During an experiment, radioactive material was released at the Oak Ridge National Laboratory in Tennessee, contaminating a significant portion of the building.

1951: The EBR-I (Experimental Breeder Reactor I) in Idaho experienced a partial meltdown during a reactor experiment, though it was contained within the facility.

1952: A power excursion at Chalk River Laboratories in Canada released radioactive water, contaminating 4,500 cubic meters of the reactor building.

1952: A criticality accident at the Argonne National Laboratory in Illinois exposed four operators to high radiation levels.

1953: A criticality accident occurred at a Russian non-reactor nuclear facility, resulting in significant radiation exposure to personnel.

1954: The Castle Bravo nuclear test on Bikini Atoll unexpectedly contaminated nearby inhabited islands and a Japanese fishing boat, exposing inhabitants and crew to radiation.

1955: A partial core meltdown occurred at the EBR-I experimental breeder reactor in Idaho, USA, though it was contained within the facility.

1955: Radioactive material was released from the Hanford nuclear reservation in Washington state, USA, contaminating a 200-mile area.

1956: During a routine maintenance operation, the Windscale Pile 1 nuclear reactor in Cumberland, England, partially melted down.

1957: The Kyshtym disaster occurred in the Soviet Union when a tank containing nuclear waste exploded, contaminating a large area and requiring the evacuation of over 10,000 people.

1957, October 10: Windscale (now Sellafield), Britain, Released 750 terabecquerels, including uranium, iodine-131, and cesium-137, during a graphite fire.

1957: Mayak Production Association, Soviet Union—An explosion released 20 million curies of strontium-90 and ruthenium isotopes.

1958: Chalk River, Canada - Radioactivity contained within the building.

1959: Santa Susana Field Laboratory, USA—A partial meltdown released radioactive gases and cesium-137, contaminating it 458 times more than the later Three Mile Island incident.

1961: Near Idaho Falls, USA - Released 80 curies of radioactivity.

1962: The Cuban Missile Crisis brought the United States and Soviet Union to the brink of nuclear war over the presence of Soviet nuclear missiles in Cuba. While not a leak or failure, this event highlighted the dangers of atomic weapons and the potential for catastrophic accidents.

1963: A criticality accident occurred at a plutonium processing facility in Siberia, resulting in the death of four workers due to acute radiation exposure.

1964: The first Chinese nuclear test, codenamed "596," was conducted at the Lop Nur test site, releasing radioactive material into the atmosphere. Although not a power plant incident, this event is relevant to nuclear-related events during this period.

1965: A partial fuel meltdown occurred at the Fermi 1 nuclear reactor near Detroit, Michigan, USA. The accident was contained within the reactor vessel, and no injuries or radioactive materials were released into the environment.

1966: Lagoona Beach (near Detroit), USA - Partial meltdown, release confined to secondary containment.

1966: Palomares, Spain - Mid-air collision contaminated 2.6 square kilometers with plutonium.

1967: A partial meltdown occurred at the Chapelcross nuclear power plant in Scotland, contaminating a portion of the reactor core.

1968, May 24: Soviet submarine K-27 experienced a reactor accident, resulting in 83 people being injured due to uneven cooling of the reactor core, causing fuel element failures and multiple ruptures.

1969, October 17: At Saint-Laurent Nuclear Power Plant in France, 50 kg of uranium dioxide melted inside the A1 reactor during a refueling operation.

1973: A chemical reaction in a process vessel at the Windscale plant in Britain released a significant amount of radioactive material.

1975: A near-core meltdown occurred at Greifswald Nuclear Power Plant in East Germany when three of six cooling water pumps were switched off for a failed test.

1975: An incident at the Leningrad Nuclear Power Plant in the Soviet Union damaged the reactor core and released radioactivity.

1976, January 5: A malfunction during fuel replacement at Jaslovské Bohunice, Czechoslovakia, resulted in fuel rod ejection from the reactor into the reactor hall by coolant.

1977: The Jaslovské Bohunice A-1 reactor in Czechoslovakia partially melted down, contaminating the reactor hall with radioactive coolant.

On November 2, 1978, Japan's first criticality accident occurred at the Fukushima No. I reactor, though this was not reported until 29 years later.

1979: Church Rock, New Mexico, USA—A dam breach released 1,100 tons of uranium tailings and 94 million gallons of contaminated wastewater into the river.

1979, March 28: Three Mile Island, USA - Released 13 to 17 curies of iodine-131 and 22 million of xenon-133.

1981: Tsuruga Nuclear Plant, Japan - Drainage released 16 tons of radioactive cooling water.

On October 17, 1981, in Buchanan, New York, USA, 100,000 gallons of water leaked into a containment building at Indian Point.

1982, January 25: Rochester, New York, USA - Steam generator leak at Ginna Nuclear Generating Station.

1983: On September 26, 1983, a significant nuclear-related incident occurred, known as the Soviet nuclear false alarm incident. The Soviet early warning system Oko erroneously reported the launch of one intercontinental ballistic missile from the United States, followed by four more. Stanislav Petrov, the duty officer at the command center, judged the warning to be a false alarm and did not relay the information up the chain of command, potentially averting a nuclear war.

1983: In November, NATO conducted a military exercise called Able Archer 83, which simulated a coordinated nuclear attack. This exercise, combined with the generally tense atmosphere of the Cold War, led to heightened Soviet alert levels and concerns about a potential NATO first strike.

1984: While not a specific incident, this year saw the continuation of cleanup and investigation efforts at Three Mile Island. In July 1984, the head of the reactor pressure vessel was removed, allowing access to the core remains from the 1979 accident. Subsequent investigation revealed that at least 45% of the core had melted.

1986, April 26: Chernobyl, Ukraine - Released 7 million curies of iodine-131, spreading contamination across Europe.

1987: Goiânia, Brazil - Abandoned radiotherapy source exposed 249 people to significant radiation from cesium-137.

1986, April 26: The Chornobyl disaster occurred in Ukraine (then part of the Soviet Union), resulting in a massive release of radioactive material. It is considered the worst nuclear accident in history.

1986, May 4: At the Hamm-Uentrop atomic power plant in West Germany, the experimental THTR-300 reactor released small amounts of fission products to the surrounding area.

1986, December 9: At the Surry Nuclear Power Plant in Virginia, USA, a feedwater pipe break killed four workers.

On March 31, 1987, Peach Bottom units 2 and 3 in Pennsylvania, USA, were shut down due to cooling malfunctions and unexplained equipment problems.

1987, December 19: Malfunctions forced the shutdown of Nine Mile Point Unit 1 in New York, USA.1989, March 28: A near core meltdown occurred at the Three Mile Island Unit 2 reactor in Pennsylvania, USA.

On April 6, 1993, a reprocessing plant at Tomsk-7 in Russia experienced an explosion in a nitric acid tank, releasing radioactive contamination.

1995, December: Tsuruga, Japan - Sodium leak at Monju Nuclear Power Plant.

1996, September 20: Seneca, Illinois, USA - Service water system failure at LaSalle Units 1 and 2.

1997, March 11: Tokaimura, Japan - Fire and explosion at nuclear reprocessing plant, 37 workers exposed to radiation.

1998: An RBMK reactor at a nuclear power plant in Saint Petersburg, Russian Federation, was shut down after a radiation leak was discovered.

1998: Worker Sergei Kharitonov revealed photographs of cracked walls and groundwater seepage at a nuclear power plant waste storage facility in Saint Petersburg,

Russian Federation. He also disclosed that the plant had been dumping 300 liters of contaminated water into the Gulf of Finland annually.

1999, June 18: Shika, Japan - Uncontrolled nuclear reaction due to mishandling of control rods.

1999, September 30: Tokaimura, Japan - Criticality accident, hundreds exposed to radiation, two workers died.

2000: The Kursk submarine disaster occurred in the Barents Sea when the Russian nuclear-powered submarine Kursk sank during a naval exercise, resulting in the deaths of all 118 crew members on board.

2000: A criticality accident occurred at the JCO uranium processing facility in Tokaimura, Japan, when workers inadvertently created a critical mass of uranium, resulting in two deaths and exposing hundreds to radiation.

2001: A small fire broke out at Germany's Philippsburg Nuclear Power Plant. It was quickly extinguished, and no radioactive material was released.

2001: An incident at the Barsebäck Nuclear Power Plant in Sweden caused a steam leak to automatically shut down one reactor, though no radiation was released.

2002: Onagawa, Japan - Two workers exposed to radiation during a fire.

2002: Davis-Besse Nuclear Power Station, Ohio, USA - Severe corrosion led to a 24-month outage.

2003: During a corrosion cleaning at the Paks Nuclear Power Plant in Hungary, fuel rods collapsed, leaking radioactive gases. The unit remained inactive for 18 months.

2003: A severe drought in France forced Électricité de France to shut down a quarter of its nuclear reactors due to the lack of cooling water from rivers.

2003: The Davis-Besse Nuclear Power Station in Oak Harbor, Ohio, USA, remained shut down for most of the year following the discovery of severe corrosion in the reactor vessel head in 2002. The plant underwent extensive repairs and upgrades.

2003: A months-long leak of highly radioactive nuclear fuel dissolved in concentrated nitric acid was discovered at the Sellafield nuclear reprocessing plant in the UK.

2004: Mihama Nuclear Power Plant, Japan - Steam explosion killed four workers and injured seven.

2005, June 16: Braidwood, Illinois, USA - Leaked tritium contaminating local water supplies.

2005, August 4: Buchanan, New York, USA - Leaked tritium and strontium into underground lakes from 1974 to 2005.

2006, March 6: Erwin, Tennessee, USA - Spilled 35 liters of highly enriched uranium.

2007: At the Kashiwazaki-Kariwa Nuclear Power Plant in Japan, a severe earthquake (measuring 6.8 on the Richter magnitude scale) caused radioactive water to spill into the Sea of Japan. All seven reactors at the plant, the world's largest single nuclear power station, were shut down for damage verification and repairs.

2007: At the Krško Nuclear Power Plant in Slovenia, a small amount of radioactive water leaked from the primary cooling circuit. The water contained within the plant did not threaten the environment or human health.

2007: At the Paks Nuclear Power Plant in Hungary, a malfunction in the cooling system of one of the reactors led to an automatic shutdown. No radiation was released, but the incident raised concerns about the plant's safety systems.

2007: A ventilation system failure at the Ascó Nuclear Power Plant in Spain released radioactive particles into the atmosphere. The incident was not reported until several months later, leading to criticism of the plant's management.

2009: November 21: Harrisburg, Pennsylvania, USA - 12 workers contaminated by radioactive dust.

2009: On December 21, 2009, an incident occurred at the Darlington Nuclear Generating Station in Ontario, Canada. More than 200,000 liters of water containing trace amounts of tritium (a radioactive isotope of hydrogen) was accidentally released into Lake Ontario. Workers mistakenly filled the wrong tank with a mixture of tritium and water.

2010: In April 2010, the Mayapuri radiological accident occurred in India. This incident resulted in one fatality after a cobalt-60 research irradiator was sold to a scrap metal dealer and dismantled.

2011: March 11: Fukushima Daiichi, Japan - Released 2.4 million curies of iodine-131 and other radionuclides following a tsunami.

2011: Marcoule Nuclear Site, France - Furnace explosion killed one person and injured four.

In 2013, at the Fukushima Daiichi Nuclear Power Plant in Japan, an open valve in the short barrier wall caused approximately 300 tonnes of contaminated water to leak from storage tanks into the surrounding area.

2013, Tepojaco, Mexico: A truck transporting a high-activity cobalt-60 teletherapy source (about 1,800 Ci or 70 TBq) was stolen near Mexico City. The source was removed from its protective shielding but remained intact. Two days later, it was recovered.

2014, Carlsbad, New Mexico, USA: Radiation was released at the Waste Isolation Pilot Plant due to an exothermic reaction in the waste drum. This did not pose a public health concern, but it did lead to improved safety protocols.

2016: Indian Point Energy Center, USA - Groundwater contamination with tritium levels reaching 14.8 million picocuries per liter.

2017: The Hanford Site in Washington, USA, experienced a structural failure, releasing radioactive debris and 56 million gallons of waste on-site.

2019: A radiation accident occurred at the State Central Navy Testing Range at Nyonoksa, near Severodvinsk, Russia, killing five military and civilian specialists.

2021: A build-up of inert gases at China's Taishan Nuclear Power Plant in Guangdong province led to concerns about a potential leak. However, no radiation release was reported outside the plant.

2022: Ukraine's Zaporizhzhia Nuclear Power Plant was shelled during the Russian invasion, causing damage to the facility and raising international concerns about nuclear safety.

2022: Russian forces seized control of the Zaporizhzhia Nuclear Power Plant in Ukraine, leading to a fire at the training complex and damage to the facility.

2022: A leak of radioactive water was discovered at the Tricastin Nuclear Power Plant in France, though officials stated it was contained within the site.

2023: A leak of tritium-contaminated water was reported at the Monticello Nuclear Generating Plant in Minnesota, USA.

2023: Japan began releasing treated radioactive water from the Fukushima Daiichi nuclear plant into the Pacific Ocean, a process expected to take decades.

2024: A 1.5 cubic meter leak of radioactive water occurred at the Fukushima Daiichi Nuclear Power Station in Japan. The leak originated from a cesium absorption tower during cleaning work.

These incidents occurred due to various factors, including equipment failure, close calls, human error, natural disasters, and design flaws. Many resulted in radioactive air, soil, and water contamination, with potential long-term environmental and health impacts. The list presented here represents only a fraction of known nuclear incidents, with many more leaks and exposures likely occurring without public knowledge or documentation. These happen daily all over the world.

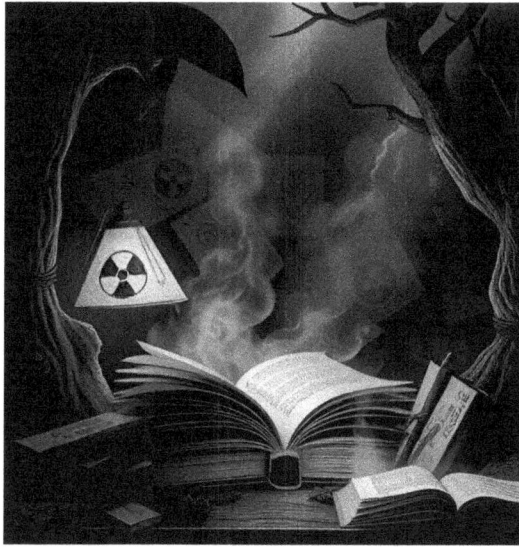

Chapter 24

Bibliography

What is Nuclear? What is Radiation?• International Atomic Energy Agency. (2020). Nuclear Power Reactors in the World. • Moore, K. (2017). The Radium Girls: The Dark Story of America's Shining Women. Sourcebooks. • Rhodes, R. (2012). The Making of the Atomic Bomb. Simon & Schuster. • U.S. Energy Information Administration. (2021). Nuclear explained. • Walker, J.S. (2004). Three Mile Island: A Nuclear Crisis in Historical

Perspective. University of California Press. • World Nuclear Association. (2021). World Uranium Mining Production. • United States Nuclear Regulatory Commission. (2020). "Radiation Basics". • International Commission on Radiological Protection. (2007). "The 2007 Recommendations of the International Commission on Radiological Protection". ICRP Publication 103. • United Nations Scientific Committee on the Effects of Atomic Radiation. (2008). "Sources and Effects of Ionizing Radiation". • World Health Organization. (2016). "Ionizing radiation, health effects, and protective measures." • Centers for Disease Control and Prevention. (2015). "Acute Radiation Syndrome: A Fact Sheet for Physicians". • National Research Council. (2006). "Health Risks from Exposure to Low Levels of Ionizing Radiation: BEIR VII Phase 2". Plus Internet Personalities Dana Dunford, Keven Blanch.

Nuclear Genesis: From Bombs to Power Plants • Beneš, P. (1999). The Environmental Impacts of Uranium Mining and Milling and the Methods of Their Reduction. • Caufield, C. (1989). Multiple Exposures: Chronicles of the Radiation Age. Harper & Row. • Groves, L.R. (1962). Now It Can Be Told: The Story of the Manhattan Project. Harper & Row. • Welcome, E. (1999). The Plutonium Files: America's Secret Medical Experiments in the Cold

War. Dial Press. Plus Internet Personalities Dana Dunford, Keven Blanch.

Unmasking the Atom's Dark Legacy • Brugge, D., & Goble, R. (2002). The history of uranium mining and the Navajo people. American Journal of Public Health, 92(9), 1410-1419. • Hacker, B. C. (1987). The Dragon's Tail: Radiation safety in the Manhattan Project, 1942-1946. University of California Press. • Kopytko, N., & Perkins, J. (2011). Climate change, nuclear power, and the adaptation–mitigation dilemma. Energy Policy, 39(1), 318-333. • Lochbaum, D. (2014). Fukushima: The Story of a Nuclear Disaster. The New Press. • Mahaffey, J. (2014). Atomic Accidents: A History of Nuclear Meltdowns and Disasters. Pegasus Books. • Medvedev, Z. A. (1990). The Legacy of Chornobyl. W. W. Norton & Company. • Perrow, C. (1999). Normal Accidents: Living with High-Risk Technologies. Princeton University Press. • Shrader-Frechette, K. (2011). What Will Work: Fighting Climate Change with Renewable Energy, Not Nuclear Power. Oxford University Press. • Sovacool, B. K. (2008). Valuing the greenhouse gas emissions from nuclear power: A critical survey. Energy Policy, 36(8), 2950-2963. • U.S. Nuclear Regulatory Commission (2020). Spent Fuel Storage in Pools and Dry Casks: Key Points and Questions & Answers. • U.S. Nuclear Regulatory Commission. (2021). License Renewal of Nuclear

Power Plants. • Weart, S. R. (2012). The Rise of Nuclear Fear. Harvard University Press. • World Nuclear Association. (2021). Nuclear Power Reactors. Plus Internet Personalities Dana Dunford, Keven Blanch.

Three Disasters That Shook the World •, Aliyu, A.S., et al. (2015). An overview of current knowledge concerning the health and environmental consequences of the Fukushima Daiichi Nuclear Power Plant (FD-NPP) accident. Environment International, 85, 213-228. • Beyea, J., et al. (2013). Accounting for long-term doses in "worldwide health effects of the Fukushima Daiichi nuclear accident." Energy & Environmental Science, 6(3), 1042-1045. • Buesseler, K.O. (2014). Fukushima and Ocean Radioactivity. Oceanography, 27(1), 92-105. • Evangeliou, N., et al. (2014). Global and local cancer risks after the Fukushima Nuclear Power Plant accident as seen from Chornobyl: A modeling study for radiocaesium (134Cs & 137Cs). Environment International, 64, 17-27. • Fukushima Prefecture. (2023). Thyroid Ultrasound Examination (Fukushima Health Management Survey). • Japan Fisheries Agency. (2023). Impact of the TEPCO's Fukushima Daiichi Nuclear Power Station accident on the fisheries industry. • Mangano, J.J., & Sherman, J.D. (2011). Elevated in vivo strontium-90 from nuclear weapons test fallout among cancer decedents: a case-control study of deciduous teeth. International Journal of Health Services, 41(1), 137-158. • Møller, A.P., & Mousseau, T.A. (2006). Biological consequences of Chernobyl: 20 years on. Trends in Ecology & Evolution, 21(4), 200-207. • Mousseau, T.A., & Møller, A.P. (2014). Genetic and Ecological Studies of Animals in Chornobyl and Fukushima. Journal of Heredity, 105(5), 704-709. • Steinhauser, G., et al. (2014). Comparison of the Chornobyl and Fukushima nuclear accidents: A review of the environmental impacts. Science of The Total Environment, 470-471, 800-817. • TEPCO. (2023). Treated Water Portal Site. • Wakeford, R. (2011). And now, Fukushima. Journal of Radiological Protection, 31(2), 167-176. • Wing, S., et al. (1997). A Reevaluation of Cancer Incidence Near the Three Mile Island Nuclear Plant. Environmental Health Perspectives, 105(1), 52-57. • World Health Organization. (2021). Fukushima Health Risk Assessment.

The Global Graveyard of Atomic Waste •, Cochran, T. B., et al. (1993). Radioactive Waste Management in the USSR: A Review of Unclassified Sources. Routledge. • Gephart, R.E. (2003). Hanford: A Conversation About Nuclear Waste and Cleanup. Battelle Press. • Lenssen, N. (1991). Nuclear Waste: The Problem that Won't Go Away. Worldwatch Institute. • Makhijani, A., et al. (1995). Nuclear Wastelands: A Global Guide to Nuclear Weapons Production and Its Health and Environmental

Effects. MIT Press. • Nikitin, M.B., et al. (2003). Wastes in the Marine Environment. Nova Science Publishers. • Olson, M. (2011). Atomic Radiation is Forever—Raven's Eye Press. • Shrader-Frechette, K. (1993). Burying Uncertainty: Risk and the Case Against Geological Disposal of Nuclear Waste. University of California Press. • Walker, J.S. (2009). The Road to Yucca Mountain: The Development of Radioactive Waste Policy in the United States. University of California Press. • Weinberg, A.M. (1994). The First Nuclear Era: The Life and Times of a Technological Fixer. AIP Press.

Nuclear Human Experiments •United States Department of Energy. (2003). "The Effects of Atomic Bombs on Health: A Review of the Literature." Retrieved from DOE. • British Medical Journal. (1955). "Radiation and Health: A Review of the Evidence." BMJ, 2(4938), 1234-1240. Retrieved from BMJ. • M. L. (2010). "The Radium Girls: They Paid with Their Lives." The New York Times. Retrieved from NYT. • Atomic Energy of Canada Limited. (2006). "Health Effects of Radiation Exposure." AECL Report. Retrieved from AECL. • United Nations Scientific Committee on the Effects of Atomic Radiation. (2008). "Report on the Chernobyl Nuclear Power Plant Accident." UNSCEAR Report 2008. Retrieved from UNSCEAR. • Medvedev, G. A. (1990). "Nuclear Disaster in the Soviet Union: The Kyshtym Accident." In Nuclear Safety and the Environment. Springer. • United States Government Accountability Office. (2004). "Nuclear Testing in the Marshall Islands: Compensation Claims and Health Effects." GAO Report, 04-1000. Retrieved from GAO. • Australian Government, Department of Health. (2015). "Health Effects of Uranium Mining." Retrieved from Health.gov.au. • Zilberman, E., & Dvornikova, E. (1994). "Ethical Violations in Soviet Medical Research." Journal of Medical Ethics, 20(1), 23-27. • French National Assembly. (2010). "Report on the Health Impact of Nuclear Tests in Algeria." Retrieved from Assemblée Nationale.

Radiation's Deadly Legacy • Cardis, E., et al. (2006). Cancer consequences of the Chornobyl accident: 20 years on. Journal of Radiological Protection, 26(2), 127-140. • Fairlie, I. (2014). A 2.2-fold excess of leukemia in young children living near German nuclear power stations. Journal of Environmental Science and Health, Part C, 32(1), 1-17. • Hatch, M., et al. (2005). Cancer in children living near nuclear power plants. BMJ, 330(7503), 1290-1291. • Koide, H. (2012). The Fukushima nuclear disaster and its effects on the environment. Global Environmental Research, 16(2), 15-24. • Kuletz, V. (1998). The Tainted Desert: Environmental and Social Ruin in the American West. Routledge. • Nussbaum, R. H. (2009). Childhood leukemia and cancers near German nuclear reactors: significance, context, and ramifications of recent studies. International Journal of Occupational and Environmental Health, 15(3), 318-323. • Pierce, D. A., et al. (1996). Studies of the mortality of atomic bomb survivors. Report 12, Part I. Cancer: 1950-1990. Radiation Research, 146(1), 1-27. • Schmitz-Feuerhake, I., et al. (2016). Genetic radiation risks: a neglected topic in the low dose debate. Environmental Health and Toxicology, 31, e2016001.

Nuclear Arsenal • Rhodes, Richard. The Making of the Atomic Bomb. Simon & Schuster, 1986.• Glasstone, Samuel, and Philip J. Dolan. The Effects of Nuclear Weapons. U.S. Department of Defense, 1977.• Walker, J. Samuel. Prompt and Utter Destruction: Truman and the Use of Atomic Bombs Against Japan. University of North Carolina Press, 2004.• Hersey, John. Hiroshima. Alfred A. Knopf, 1946.• Weisgall, Jonathan M. Operation Crossroads: The Atomic Tests at Bikini Atoll. Naval Institute Press, 1994.• Arms Control Association. (2024). Treaties & Agreements. • Atomic Archive. (n.d.). Nuclear Testing Chronology. • Britannica. (n.d.). Arms control | Nuclear Disarmament, Treaty Negotiations. • Hiroshima for Peace. (2024). The status of nuclear forces (estimated as of January 2024). • International Campaign to Abolish Nuclear Weapons. (2024). Countries with nuclear weapons. • NATO. (2023, February 27). Arms control, disarmament, and nonproliferation in NATO. • SIPRI.

(2024, June 17). The role of nuclear weapons grows as geopolitical relations deteriorate: The new SIPRI Yearbook is out now. • United Nations Office for Disarmament Affairs. (n.d.). Treaty on the Nonproliferation of Nuclear Weapons (NPT). • World Population Review. (2024). Nuclear Weapons by Country 2024.• Schlosser, Eric. Command and Control: Nuclear Weapons, the Damascus Accident, and the Illusion of Safety. Penguin Books, 2013.• Cirincione, Joseph. Bomb Scare: The History and Future of Nuclear Weapons. Columbia University Press, 2007.• Federation of American Scientists. (2024). Status of World Nuclear Forces.• Stockholm International Peace Research Institute. (2024). SIPRI Yearbook: Armaments, Disarmament, and International Security.• Bulletin of the Atomic Scientists. (2024). Nuclear Notebook. Flora Lewis, "The Broken Arrow: The Accidental Bombing of Spain," The Atlantic • Tad Szulc, "H-Bomb Lost in Spain in 1966 Mishap," The New York Times • U.S. Department of Defense, "Narrative Summaries of Accidents Involving U.S. Nuclear Weapons, 1950-1980" • Spanish Nuclear Safety Council, "Palomares Follow-up Program"

The Razor's Edge: • BBC News. (2013, September 26), Stanislav Petrov: The man who may have saved the world • Bradshaw, M. (2017). 1983 Nuclear False Alarm. Stanford University • National Security Archive. (2012,

March 1). The 3 A.M. Phone Call: False Missile Attack Warning Incidents, 1979-1980 • Wikipedia. (2024, November 21). 1961 Goldsboro B-52 crash • Super Sabre Society. (n.d.). Today in History - March 11, 1958 - B-47 accidentally drops a nuclear bomb on a house in Mars Bluff, SC • Wikipedia. (2024, November 12). 1983 Soviet nuclear false alarm incident • PBS. (n.d.). Russia's Nuclear Warriors | False Alarms on the Nuclear Front • Center for Arms Control and Nonproliferation. (2022, October 14). The Goldsboro B-52 Crash • Wikipedia. (2024, December 2). 1958 Mars Bluff B-47 nuclear weapon loss incident • Center for Arms Control and Nonproliferation. (2022, October 14). The Soviet False Alarm Incident and Able Archer 83 • PBS. (n.d.). Russia's Nuclear Warriors | False Alarms on the Nuclear Front • Center for Arms Control and Nonproliferation. (2022, October 14). The Soviet False Alarm Incident and Able Archer 83 • National Security Archive. (2012, March 1). The 3 A.M. Phone Call: False Missile Attack Warning Incidents, 1979-1980 • Wikipedia. (2024, November 12). 1983 Soviet nuclear false alarm incident • BBC News. (2013, September 26). Stanislav Petrov: The man who may have saved the world

Tritium• Centers for Disease Control and Prevention. (n.d.). Prescription Drug Use in the United States. • Environmental Protection Agency. (2022). Radionuclides in Drinking Water. • European Commission. (2020). Directive on the Quality of Water Intended for Human Consumption. • Health Physics Society. (2022). Tritium Fact Sheet. • International Atomic Energy Agency. (2022). Tritium and the Environment. • Journal of Environmental Radioactivity. (2019). Tritium in the Aquatic Environment. • National Research Council. (2006). Health Risks from Exposure to Low Levels of Ionizing Radiation: BEIR VII Phase 2. • Nuclear Energy Institute. (2023). Nuclear Plant Tritium Releases. • Nuclear Regulatory Commission. (2021). Tritium, Radiation Protection Limits, and Drinking Water Standards. • U.S. Geological Survey. (2021). Tritium in Groundwater Near Nuclear Facilities. • World Health Organization. (n.d.). Pharmaceuticals in Drinking Water. • World Nuclear Association. (2023). Radioisotopes in Industry.

Radioactive Water• Eerkes-Medrano, D., Thompson, R .C., & Aldridge, D.C. (2016). Microplastics in Freshwater Systems: A Review of the Emerging Threats. Environmental Pollution, 218, 1045-1059. • Grand View Research. (2022). Bottled Water Market Size, Share & Trends Analysis Report By Product, Region, And Segment Forecasts, 2022 - 2030. • LaMotte, S. (2024, January 8). Bottled Water May Contain High Levels of Nanoplastics, Study Finds. CNN Health.

Fires Unintended Consequence • Ager, A.A., et al. (2019). The wildfire problem in areas contaminated by the Chornobyl disaster. Science of The Total Environment, 696, 133954.• Evangeliou, N., et al. (2014). Wildfires in Chernobyl-contaminated forests and risks to the population and the environment: A new nuclear disaster about to happen? Environment International, 73, 346-358.• Evangeliou, N., et al. (2016). Resuspension and atmospheric transport of radionuclides due to wildfires near the Chornobyl Nuclear Power Plant in 2015: An impact assessment. Scientific Reports, 6, 26062.• Kalinina-Pohl, M., et al. (2020). Assessing Fire Damage in the Chornobyl Exclusion Zone. James Martin Center for Nonproliferation Studies.• Kovalevskaya, L. (2020). Chornobyl still burns - Greenpeace International. Greenpeace.org.

Nuclear Submarines • Wilkinson, E. P. (1955). "Nautilus 90 North". World Publishing Company. • Clancy, T. (1993). "Submarine: A Guided Tour Inside a Nuclear Warship". Berkley. • Polmar, N., & Moore, K. J. (2004). "Cold War Submarines: The Design and Construction of U.S. and Soviet Submarines". Potomac Books. • Nilsen, T., Kudrik, I., & Nikitin, A. (1996). "The Russian Northern Fleet: Sources of Radioactive Contamination". Bellona Foundation. • Handler, J. (1995). "The Russian Fleet's Nuclear Submarine Accidents." Jane's Intelligence Review.

• Høibråten, S., Thoresen, P. E., & Haugan, A. (2003). "The environmental impact of the sunken submarine Komsomolets." Norwegian Defence Research Establishment. • Reistad, O., & Ølgaard, P. L. (2006). "Inventory and Source Term Evaluation of Russian Nuclear Submarines." Nordic Nuclear Safety Research. • Kristensen, H. M., & Korda, M. (2021). "Nuclear Notebook: How many nuclear weapons does Russia have in 2021?". Bulletin of the Atomic Scientists. • Bukharin, O., & Handler, J. (1995). "Russian Nuclear-Powered Submarine Decommissioning". Science & Global Security. • International Atomic Energy Agency. (2001). "Inventory of accidents and losses at sea involving radioactive material." IAEA-TECDOC-1242.

Censorship, Compartmentalization, Secrecy • Atomic Heritage Foundation. (2019). Manhattan Project. • Bulletin of the Atomic Scientists. (2021). Nuclear Notebook. • Environmental Protection Agency. (2021). Radiation Protection. • Greenpeace. (2019). The Global Crisis of Nuclear Waste. • International Atomic Energy Agency. (2020). Chornobyl: The True Scale of the Accident. • Nuclear Energy Institute. (2021). Nuclear Energy in the U.S. • Stockholm International Peace Research Institute. (2020). World Nuclear Forces. • Union of Concerned Scientists. (2018). The Nuclear Power Dilemma. • World Health Organization. (2020). Ionizing Radiation, Health

Effects and Protective Measures. • World Nuclear Association. (2021). Fukushima Daiichi Accident.

Radon • Environmental Protection Agency. "A Citizen's Guide to Radon." EPA.gov, 2016. • National Research Council. "Health Effects of Exposure to Radon: BEIR VI." National Academies Press, 1999. • World Health Organization. "WHO Handbook on Indoor Radon: A Public Health Perspective." WHO.int, 2009. • Agency for Toxic Substances and Disease Registry. "Toxicological Profile for Radon." ATSDR.CDC.gov, 2012. • National Cancer Institute. "Radon and Cancer." Cancer.gov, 2011.

The Radioactive Waste Is Piling Up• Arms Control Association. (2023). Nuclear Weapons: Who Has What at a Glance. • Federation of American Scientists. (2024). Status of World Nuclear Forces.

Fighting Cancer With Cancer • Centers for Disease Control and Prevention. (2022). Health Effects of Radiation. • Environmental Protection Agency. (2023). Radiation Protection. • Greenpeace. (2023). The True Cost of Nuclear Power. • International Agency for Research on Cancer. (2021). World Cancer Report. • International Atomic Energy Agency. (2023). Nuclear Safety and Security. • National Cancer Institute. (2023). Cancer Trends Progress Report. • Nuclear Regulatory Commission. (2024). Radioactive Waste Management. • Union of

Concerned Scientists. (2024). Nuclear Power and Public Health. • United Nations Scientific Committee on the Effects of Atomic Radiation. (2022). Sources and Effects of Ionizing Radiation. • World Health Organization. (2024). Global Cancer Statistics. • Reddit. (2021, November 26). Eben Byers: The Man Who Drank Radioactive Water Until His Jaw Fell Off. r/Damnthatsinteresting. Retrieved November 15, 2024.• Reddit. (2021, July 27). Is it safe to bathe in a radium/radon hot spring? r/Radiation. Retrieved November 15, 2024.• Wikipedia. (n.d.). Ciudad Juárez cobalt-60 contamination incident. Retrieved November 15, 2024.• Peng, L., Yang, B., Lai, X., et al. (2020). Effects of Radon From Hot Springs on Lymphocyte Subsets in Peripheral Blood. Dose-Response, 18(1). Published January-March 2020.• Wikipedia. (n. d.). Goiânia accident. Retrieved November 15, 2024.• Britannica. (2024, October 28). Goiania accident (1987). Retrieved November 15, 2024.• Johnston, W. R. (2008, October 26). Mexico City orphaned source, 1962. Johnston's Archive. Retrieved November 15, 2024.• Instadose. (2018, July 19). The Dangers of Shoe-Fitting Fluoroscopes. Retrieved November 15, 2024.• The Vintage News. (2023, June 29). The 1962 Radioactive Disaster in Mexico City That Destroyed a Family. Retrieved November 15, 2024.from https://www.madeinchicagomuseum.com/single-post/westclox/• RIVM. (2017, August 31). Electromagnetic fields in daily life. Retrieved November 15, 2024, from https://www.rivm.nl/en/electro-magnetic-fields/emf-dailylife

Radioactive Milk Testing • Brown, K. (2013). Plutopia: Nuclear Families, Atomic Cities, and the Great Soviet and American Plutonium Disasters. Oxford University Press. • Caldicott, H. (2014). Crisis Without End: The Medical and Ecological Consequences of the Fukushima Nuclear Catastrophe. The New Press. • Nadesan, M. H. (2013). Fukushima and the Privatization of Risk. Palgrave Macmillan. • Perrow, C. (2011). The Next Catastrophe: Reducing Our Vulnerabilities to Natural, Industrial, and Terrorist Disasters. Princeton University Press. • Steinhauser, G., Brandl, A., & Johnson, T. E. (2014). Comparison of the Chornobyl and Fukushima nuclear accidents: A review of the environmental impacts. Science of The Total Environment, 470-471, 800-817

World Without Compassion: Governments' Disregard for Nuclear Testing Victims •Wikipedia. "Semipalatinsk Test Site." Accessed December 16, 2024. https://en.wikipedia.org/wiki/Semipalatinsk_Test_Site • United Nations General Assembly. "Document A/78/312: International cooperation and coordination for the human and ecological rehabilitation and economic development of the Semipalatinsk region of Kazakhstan." August 16, 2023. • Grosche, B., et al. "Studies of health effects from nuclear testing near the Semipalatinsk Nuclear Test Site, Kazakhstan." Central Asian Journal of Global Health, August 29, 2019. https://www.ncbi.nlm.nih.gov/pmc/articles/PMC6734094/ • International Atomic Energy Agency. "Semipalatinsk Revisited." IAEA Bulletin, 40/4/1998. https://www.iaea.org/sites/default/files/publications/magazines/bulletin/bull40-4/4040508121 • Parfitt, T. "The legacy of Semipalatinsk nuclear testing: A cautionary tale." The Lancet EClinicalMedicine, 2019. • Kassenova, T. "Banning Nuclear Testing: Lessons From the Semipalatinsk Nuclear Testing Site." Carnegie Endowment for International Peace, March 10, 2017. https://carnegieendowment.org/2017/03/10/banning-nuclear-testing-lessons-from-semipalatinsk-nuclear-testing-site-pub-68218 • Nuclear Threat Initiative. "Semipalatinsk Test Site." Accessed December 16, 2024. https://www.nti.org/education-center/facilities/semipalatinsk-test-site • Kassenova, T. "Atomic Steppe: How Kazakhstan Gave Up the Bomb." Carnegie Endowment for International Peace, February 5, 2022. https://carnegieendowment.org/2022/02/05/atomic-steppe-how-kazakhstan-gave-up-bomb-pub-86350• "Embittered City" (documentary) • Nevada-Semipalatinsk Movement records • Soviet nuclear testing archives • Navajo Nation health studies • Semipalatinsk Test Site research papers

• Yunkom Mine historical documents • Kazakhstan environmental impact reports • US government uranium mining records • World Health Organization radiation exposure data • International Atomic Energy Agency reports

Radioactive Scrap in Our Everyday Lives • Acerinox incident in Spain (1998) • Ayutthaya Province, Thailand incident (2008) • Chachoengsao Province, Thailand incident (2008) • Ciudad Juárez, Mexico incident (1983) • Goiânia accident in Brazil (1987) • Henan Province, China incident (1999) • IAEA Incident and Trafficking Database (ITDB) • Istanbul, Turkey incident (1998-1999) • Jilin, China incident (1996) • Kingisepp, Russia incident (1999) • Kola Harbor, Russia incident (2003) • Mayapuri incident in India (2010) • Ohio and Pennsylvania, USA incident (2016) • Samut Prakan, Thailand incident (2000) • Shaanxi Province, China incident (2009) • The Polygon, Kazakhstan • Tianjin Hongdi Engineering Inspection Development Co. incident in Nanjing, China (2014) • Vicente Sotelo Alardín and Ricardo Hernández's involvement in the Ciudad Juárez incident • Yanango incident in Peru (1999) • Yunkom Mine, Ukraine

The Next Extinction Event • American Cancer Society. (2024). Cancer Facts & Figures.• Centers for Disease Control and Prevention. (2023). National Vital Statistics Reports.• International Commission on Radiological Protection. (2022). Occupational Intakes of Radionu-clides.• Journal of Environmental Radioactivity. (2023). Special Issue: Radioactive Contamination in Marine En-vironments.• Nature. (2022). Temporal Trends in Sperm Count: A Systematic Review and Meta-Regression Analy-sis.• Science. (2021). Long-term Ecological Impacts of Nuclear Accidents.• The Lancet. (2023). Global Burden of Disease Study.

We Now Eat Radioactive Food •Food and Agricul-ture Organization of the United Nations (FAO), In-ternational Atomic Energy Agency (IAEA), and World Health Organization (WHO), "Criteria for Radionuclide Activity Concentrations for Food and Drinking Water," IAEA-TECDOC-1788, Vienna, 2016 •Environmental Pro-tection Agency (EPA), "Radionuclides in Drinking Wa-ter," Washington, D.C., 2000 •World Health Organiza-tion (WHO), "Guidelines for Drinking-water Quality, 4th Edition," Geneva, 2011• International Commission on Radiological Protection (ICRP), "Age-dependent Doses to Members of the Public from Intake of Radionu-clides - Part 5 Compilation of Ingestion and Inhalation Dose Coefficients," ICRP Publication 72, Oxford, 1996 •United Nations Scientific Committee on the Effects of Atomic Radiation (UNSCEAR), "Sources and Effects of Ionizing Radiation," New York, 2008 •National Coun-cil on Radiation Protection and Measurements (NCRP),

"Ionizing Radiation Exposure of the Population of the United States," NCRP Report No. 160, Bethesda, MD, 2009 •Codex Alimentarius Commission, "General Standard for Contaminants and Toxins in Food and Feed," CXS 193-1995, Rome, 2019• International Atomic Energy Agency (IAEA), "Measurement of Radionuclides in Food and the Environment," Technical Reports Series No. 295, Vienna, 1989• U.S. Food and Drug Administration (FDA), "Compliance Policy Guide Sec. 560.750 Radionuclides in Imported Foods - Levels of Concern," Silver Spring, MD, 2005 • European Commission, "Council Regulation (Euratom) 2016/52 laying down maximum permitted levels of radioactive contamination of food and feed following a nuclear accident or any other case of radiological emergency," Brussels, 2016

Nuclear Power Plant Leaks the Shortlist • Alexievich, S. (2006). Voices from Chernobyl: The Oral History of a Nuclear Disaster. Picador. • Busby, C. (2011). Fukushima and Health: What to Expect. Green Audit Press. • Gale, R. P., & Lax, E. (2013). Radiation: What It Is, What You Need to Know. Knopf. • Johnston, B. R. (2007). Half-lives and Half-truths: Confronting the Radioactive Legacies of the Cold War. School for Advanced Research Press.

The Global Nuclear Pollution Players • Atomic Energy Commission Report CF-169 "Investigation of Radiation Incident at the Westinghouse Testing Reactor, License Number TR-2, Waltz Mill, Pennsylvania", dated May 27, 1960. • Westinghouse Report WTR-49, Report on WTR Fuel Element Failure of April 3, 1960. • "Radioactive Leaks Found at Reactors," Chemical & Engineering News, 2006. • "Probe Finds Ongoing Radioactive Leaks at Illinois Nuclear Plants," Voice of America, 2017. • "Fact Sheet: Nuclear Proliferation Risks in Nuclear Energy Programs," Center for Arms Control and Nonproliferation, updated March 2021. • NuScale Power official website, accessed 2024. • TerraPower official website, Natrium technology page, accessed 2024. • Wikipedia, "General Electric," accessed 2024. • Westinghouse Nuclear official website, accessed 2024. • National Cancer Institute, "Accidents at Nuclear Power Plants and Cancer Risk," updated May 12, 2022. • World Nuclear Association, "Outline History of Nuclear Energy," updated August 29, 2024. • Friends of the Earth Australia, "The Global Uranium Industry & Cameco's Troubled History," May 13, 2017. • Chemical & Engineering News, "Radioactive Leaks Found At Reactors," June 26, 2006. • Wikipedia, "Environmental impact of nuclear power," accessed 2024. • Friends of the Earth, "Is Nuclear Power Bad for the Environment?", accessed 2024.

Additional Resources for above chapters • Brown, K. (2013). Plutopia: Nuclear Families, Atomic Cities, and the Great Soviet and American Plutonium Disasters. Oxford

University Press. • Fuller, J.G. (1975). We Almost Lost Detroit—Reader's Digest Press. • Medvedev, Z.A. (1979). Nuclear Disaster in the Urals. W.W. Norton & Company. • Simon, S.L. et al. (2010). Radiation Doses and Cancer Risks in the Marshall Islands Associated with Exposure to Radioactive Fallout from Bikini and Enewetak Nuclear Weapons Tests. Health Physics, 99(2), 105-123. • Sovacool, B.K. (2011). Contesting the Future of Nuclear Power. World Scientific. • Stacy, S. (2000). Proving the Principle: A History of the Idaho National Engineering and Environmental Laboratory, 1949-1999. U.S. Department of Energy.

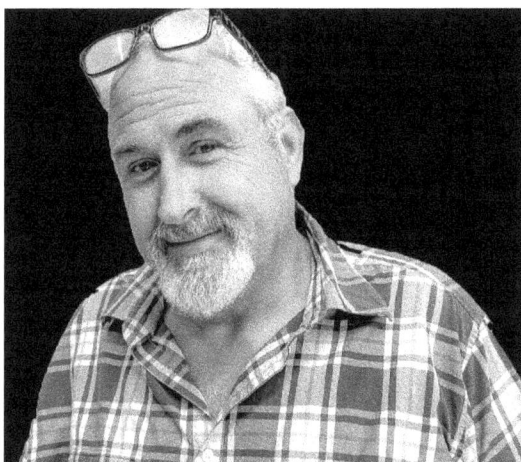

Chapter 25

Further Reading Books By Marko Vovk On Amazon Books

Hey there! I'm thrilled to share my journey into book publishing with you. After semi-retiring and weathering the storm of COVID-19, I've discovered a new passion that's set my creative spirit on fire! Now, I'll be the first to admit I'm no English major or fiction virtuoso. But what I lack in literary prowess, I make up for with a treasure trove of education, knowledge, and real-world experiences. Plus, I've got research skills that would make a detective jealous!

Each book I craft is a labor of love, penned by you honestly, with a bit of help from some nifty editing software. I even design my covers—talk about wearing multiple hats! Regarding publishing, I'm proudly independent, embracing the self-publishing route.

I will tell you a secret: my writing has been quite the journey. With each book, I feel like I'm leveling up and honing my craft. While I may not be gunning for a spot on The New York Times bestseller list (yet!), my books are bursting at the seams with information.

Here's the beauty of my books – you can dive in from any chapter and still strike gold. Fair warning, though: I pack in information like I'm preparing for an intellectual apocalypse. And yes, my experiences and beliefs might color the pages a bit. But hey, that's what makes them uniquely mine.

I always encourage my readers to treat my books as a springboard for exploration. Dive deeper, question everything, and forge your path to the truth. Sometimes, I might get a tad carried away and exaggerate a concept or two—it's all part of my charm! I'm eager to hear from my readers. Do you have suggestions or ideas for improvements? Please shoot me an email! Thanks to the magic of Amazon KDP, I can tweak and update faster than you can say "revised edition."

As we wrap up 2024, I'm proud to look back at the books I've published over the past two years. It's been a wild ride, and I can't wait to see what literary adventures await in the coming year! Remember, if you're looking for a no-nonsense, information-packed read with a dash of personal flair, you've come to the right place. Happy reading, and here's to the joy of lifelong learning!

1. Avoid Waterproofing, Drain Cleaning and Foundation Repair Scams

2. Childless Cat Lady: Movement, Dynamics, Health, and Political Influence

3. Make Your Home Great Again

4. Deep Down The Rabbit Hole Poetry

5. Don't Rent this Home, Condo, or Apartment

6. Fix Your Toxic Home and Live Longer

7. Nuclear Extinction Event Is Killing Our Families

8. Pets: The Hidden Costs of Companionship

9. Project 2025 Quick Review

10. The Water You Drink May Be Killing You

www.ingramcontent.com/pod-product-compliance
Lightning Source LLC
Chambersburg PA
CBHW070800280326

41934CB00012B/2998